Practical Fibreoptic Intubation

To my wife, Anju for her support and encouragement and to our sons, Hemal and Bhavesh, for their patience and understanding

Senior commissioning editor: Melanie Tait
Development editor: Zoë Youd
Production controller: Chris Jarvis
Desk editor: Claire Hutchins
Cover designer: Fred Rose

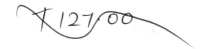

Practical Fibreoptic Intubation

Mansukh Popat MBBS FRCA

Consultant Anaesthetist
Nuffield Department of Anaesthetics
Oxford Radcliffe Hospitals NHS Trust
Oxford
UK

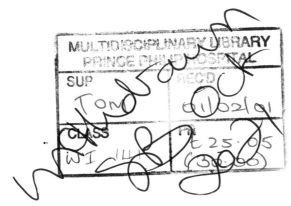
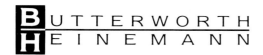

BUTTERWORTH
HEINEMANN

OXFORD   AUCKLAND   BOSTON   JOHANNESBURG   MELBOURNE   NEW DELHI

Butterworth-Heinemann
Linacre House, Jordan Hill, Oxford OX2 8DP
225 Wildwood Avenue, Woburn, MA 01801-2041
A division of Reed Educational and Professional Publishing Ltd

A member of the Reed Elsevier plc group

First published 2001

© Reed Educational and Professional Publishing Ltd 2001

British Library Cataloguing in Publication Data
A catalogue record for this book is available from the British Library

Library of Congress Cataloging in Publication Data
A catalogue record for this book is available from the Library of Congress

ISBN 0 7506 4496 6

Composition by Genesis Typesetting, Laser Quay, Rochester, Kent
Printed and bound in Spain by Artes Graficas Elkar, Bizkaia

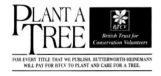

Contents

Foreword

This book was needed. The literature on fibreoptic techniques is extensive, many interesting and useful techniques have been described, and I would be surprised if the most experienced endoscopist did not find something new here. The labour of collating and illustrating all this information must have been formidable. I salute and am grateful for Dr Popat and his colleagues' energy and enthusiasm.

Flexible fibreoptic technology allows today's anaesthetists to deal calmly with pathology that would have sorely tried, or even defeated, our less fortunate predecessors. However, the learning curve can be shallow if experienced tuition is not available. Anyone who has read this book will steepen his or her learning curve dramatically. Dr Popat's observation that successful endoscopy is 'in the mind' of the endoscopist rings very true to me. Novice endoscopists, who take the trouble to prepare their minds by reading this book, will need little further instruction.

Dr Popat is careful to point out that flexible fibreoptic techniques are unsuitable in an important minority of patients. Choosing the right technique, rather than the most technologically up to date one, is the mark of experience. Nevertheless, I feel certain that practitioners who have mastered the fibrescope sleep better at night. If you can't do it, you should buy this book.

Ian Calder
Consultant Anaesthetist
The National Hospital for Neurology and Neurosurgery
and
Royal Free Hospital, London, UK

Preface

Flexible fibreoptic endoscopy and intubation has revolutionized airway management in recent years. It is a skill that is not only useful in safely intubating a patient with a difficult airway but has many other applications in anaesthesia and intensive care. It is therefore not surprising that every anaesthetist wants to become skilled in using fibreoptic instruments.

The goal of this book is to prepare the reader in performing the skill of fibreoptic techniques to its fullest extent with the highest degree of success. I believe that a structured learning process and thorough understanding of the practical aspects of fibreoptic techniques is required to achieve this goal.

Some fundamental aspects of fibreoptic equipment, learning basic endoscopy skills and the role of fibreoptic intubation in difficult airway management are covered first as part of a structured learning process.

Detailed description of fibreoptic intubation techniques in the anaesthetized and awake patient, including the paediatrics follow. Causes of difficulties in fibreoptic intubation and their practical solutions are given, as are techniques for uses other than intubation described. All the practical procedures are described in a step-by-step manner with many photographs and endoscopy images reinforcing the text.

This book is intended to form a ready source of practical advice to anaesthetists of all grades contemplating using fibreoptic intubation techniques. It will also be useful to other specialists such as intensivists and accident and emergency physicians involved in airway management. Trainers in fibreoptic intubation will find plenty of advice on teaching techniques and the fully referenced text will form a foundation for preparing tutorials and lectures.

Acknowledgements

The idea of writing this book follows the success of fibreoptic intubation training in my department in Oxford and the many practical workshops that we organize to teach others. I am indebted to all the individuals who include not only anaesthetic colleagues but also anaesthetic assistants and surgeons who have put in an enormous amount of hard work and dedication. Dr Atul Kapila and Dr Stuart Benham have been splendid partners in organizing the teaching and have co-authored a chapter each and reviewed the text in this book. I would like to give special thanks to my friend and colleague, Mr Stephen Watt-Smith, Consultant Maxillofacial Surgeon, for his constant support and encouragement in my commitment to teaching and training.

I am grateful to KeyMed Ltd for providing the flexible fibreoptic endoscopy and video equipment used for taking endoscopy images for this book. The constant support of their many personnel over the years is very much appreciated.

All the artwork, including that for the cover design of the book, photographs and editing of endoscopy images was done by staff at the Oxford Medical Illustration department. I appreciate their enthusiastic and energetic approach in finishing the work in time.

The editorial and production team of Butterworth-Heinemann deserve a special mention for the timely production of the book.

Mrs Pat Millard spent hours on the computer with the manuscript and I wish to acknowledge her constant support.

Mansukh Popat

1

Fibreoptic endoscopy equipment

- History and development of flexible fibrescopes
- Physics of light transmission through a fibreoptic bundle
- Parts of an adult intubating fibrescope
- Light sources, camera and monitor
- Care, cleaning and disinfection of fibreoptic equipment
- Checking fibreoptic equipment
- Choice of flexible fibrescopes

● History and development of flexible fibrescopes

The quest for methods to examine the internal structure and working of the human body without resorting to surgery has been a major challenge for many centuries. Two factors, the flexibility and illumination of instruments, restricted their potential. In 1927, John L. Baird, a British scientist, took out a patent on a method he had discovered for transmitting light along flexible glass bundles. The optical quality of his system was poor and it was not until 1954 that Hopkins and Kapany from Imperial College, London, announced the construction of a coherent bundle of flexible glass fibres capable of transmitting a clear, sharp image [1]. Four years later, Hirschowitz and colleagues in Michigan, USA [2], developed the first prototype of a fully functional flexible fibregastroscope. This event marked the beginning of the era of the use of flexible fibreoptic instruments in medicine.

In 1967, Dr Peter Murphy, then a Senior Anaesthetic Registrar at the National Hospital for Neurology and Neurosurgery at Queen Square in London, described the first fibreoptic-guided tracheal intubation in anaesthetized patients [3]. He was inspired by the description, in *The Lancet*, of a flexible choledochoscope to view the inside of bile ducts and used a similar instrument. The first bronchofibrescope was developed in 1968 and two years later Ikeda from Japan presented its use in 100 patients with lung cancer[4]. In 1972, Taylor and Towey (UK) described the use of a bronchofibrescope to intubate patients 'awake'[5]. A few weeks later, Conyers and colleagues (Canada) described the use of a bronchofibrescope for awake intubation in a patient with rheumatoid arthritis[6]. In the same year Stiles and colleagues, using a dedicated fibreoptic laryngoscope, reported a series of 100 cases with a 96% success rate[7]. In 1973, Davis described the use of a dedicated fibreoptic laryngoscope for awake intubation in a patient with ankylosing spondylitis[8]. A similar instrument was used by Prithvi Raj and co-workers in 50 patients[9]. These earlier instruments were less expensive and light could be supplied with an external fibreoptic illuminator or by a snap-on battery handle, but the insertion cord was short (Figure 1.1a).

The new generation of flexible intubating fibreoptic laryngoscopes was introduced in the mid-1980s, one of the first being the LF-1 (Olympus, Japan). The insertion cord was made 60 cm long so that a tracheal tube could be mounted on it with enough length still available to gain access to the trachea before 'railroading' would start (Figure 1.1b). The insertion cord was also made more robust to withstand the forces of railroading a tracheal tube, and its diameter was reduced to 4 mm to allow tracheal tubes of 5 mm and larger to easily pass over it. Currently, fibrescopes made by different manufacturers are available for use in a wide range of applications in anaesthesia and intensive care.

● Physics of light transmission through a fibreoptic bundle

When light travels from one medium to another, e.g. from air to glass, depending on the angle of incidence, some of it is transmitted, some is absorbed and the rest is reflected internally. When glass is heated and stretched, the resultant glass fibre can be so arranged that light from an object at one end of the glass fibre can be internally reflected along the length of the fibre and exit at the other end and still retain a sharp image of the original object. If many such fibres are grouped together to form a '**flexible bundle**', the size and clarity of image transmission can be built up to become clinically useful. A typical flexible bundle

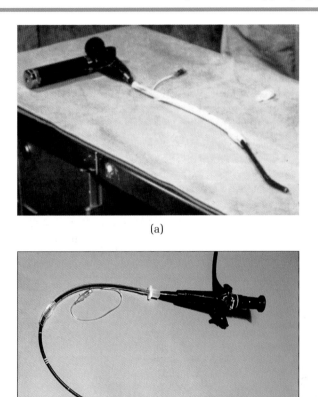

(a)

(b)

Figure 1.1 (a) A dedicated fibreoptic laryngoscope used in 1974. Note the short insertion cord (From Prithvi Raj *et al.* [9] with permission from Lippincott, Williams and Wilkins). (b) A modern intubating fibreoptic laryngoscope (Olympus LF-2). The long insertion cord allows a tracheal tube to be mounted on it with enough length available to gain access to the trachea before railroading starts

contains 10 000 glass fibres, each of 8–10 μm diameter. To reduce the amount of light leaking out of the fibres due to refraction, each individual fibre is covered with another thin film (1 μm) of glass by a process called **cladding**. The fibres in a bundle are arranged in a specific manner such that the arrangement is the same at both ends of the fibreoptic bundle. This is called a **coherent or image transmitting bundle**. The transmitted image is a composite of the small portions formed by each fibre akin to the picture formed on a television screen. The fibreoptic bundles transmitting light from the light source to the object are not specifically arranged and are called **incoherent or light transmission bundles**.

The light transmission and image formation in a flexible intubating fibrescope is very simply explained in Figure 1.2. Light from an external light source travels via light transmission (incoherent) fibreoptic bundles to the distal end of the fibrescope and illuminates the object. The light from the object is reflected onto the objective lens at the tip of the fibrescope. The objective lens focuses the light onto the image transmission (coherent)

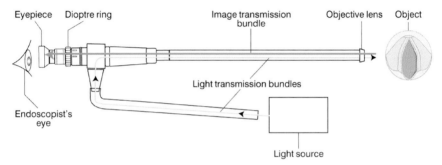

Figure 1.2 Simplified representation of light transmission and image formation in a flexible intubating fibrescope

bundle, through which it is internally reflected. The image, which is a composite of lots of small spots of light, each with uniform intensity and colour from each fibre, is reconstructed in the eyepiece at the proximal end of the fibrescope. The image can then be focused onto the viewer's retina by a dioptre ring so that it is sharp.

● Parts of an adult intubating fibrescope (e.g. Olympus LF-2)

The intubating fibrescope consists of the following parts (Figure 1.3):

> **Body**
> **Insertion cord**
> **Universal light cord**

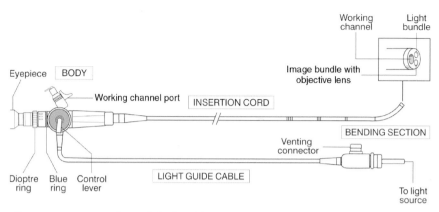

Figure 1.3   Parts of an adult flexible intubating fibrescope
(e.g. Olympus FL-2)

Body

The shape of the body allows the fibrescope to be held
comfortably in the palm of either hand. The thumb of the same
hand is used to manipulate the control lever and the index finger
to activate the working channel. The conical connection between
the body and the insertion cord facilitates loading of a tracheal
tube. The blue ring on the body signifies that the whole of the
fibrescope can safely be immersed in a disinfectant. The body
has the following parts:

> **Control lever**
> **Eyepiece and dioptre ring**
> **Working channel port**

Control lever

The control lever moves the tip of the fibrescope in a vertical
plane only by activating angulation wires in the insertion cord.
When the control lever is pressed down, the tip faces anteriorly
and when the control lever is moved up, the tip points
posteriorly.

Eyepiece and dioptre ring

The eyepiece is made up of several lenses and collects the
composite image from the fibres in the image transmission
fibreoptic bundle. The dioptre ring can be adjusted so that a

sharp image is focused on the retina of the operator. When viewed in the eyepiece, a pointer is seen which is an 'orientation mark'. This mark helps in orientating the operator to the anterior direction of the tip.

Working channel port

The working channel port incorporates the suction connector and a valve that is covered by a rubber cap. The port is connected to the distal end of the fibrescope through the working channel in the insertion cord. The port can be used for suction, instillation of drugs and oxygen, and insertion of wires for anterograde and retrograde fibreoptic intubation techniques. The spring-loaded suction valve is activated when it is pressed by the index finger.

Insertion cord

This is the part of the fibrescope that is advanced into the trachea and acts as the flexible guide for railroading the tracheal tube to facilitate intubation. Its outer diameter determines the size of the smallest tracheal tube that can easily be passed over it. This is usually 1 mm greater than the diameter of the insertion cord; for example, the Olympus LF-2 fibrescope with insertion cord diameter of 4 mm will allow a tracheal tube of 5 mm or larger to easily pass over it. It is 60 cm long, allowing railroading to begin after its tip is positioned in the trachea. There are white indicators every 5 cm from 15 to 40 cm. The insertion cord has the following parts (Figure 1.4):

> **Image transmission bundle (coherent bundle)**
> **Light transmission bundles (incoherent bundles)**
> **Working channel**
> **Angulation wires and distal bending section**

These parts are tightly wrapped in a watertight plastic casing, making the insertion cord robust but flexible enough to facilitate railroading of a tracheal tube.

Image transmission bundle

The physics of the image transmission bundle has already been discussed. There are about 6000 fibres in this bundle.

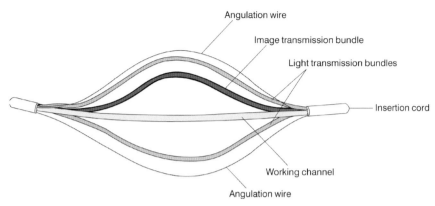

Figure 1.4   Parts of the insertion cord of an Olympus LF-2 intubating fibrescope

Light transmission bundles

These are two bundles carrying light from the light source to the object.

Working channel

The working channel extends proximally from the working channel port in the body of the fibrescope to the tip at its distal end. It is enclosed in a plastic casing, preventing fluid entering the fibreoptic bundles. The working channel facilitates suction, instillation of drugs and oxygen and passage of guide wires. The power of the suction depends on the diameter of this channel. An Olympus LF-2 fibrescope has a 1.5 mm channel, which is just adequate but not very powerful.

Angulation wires and distal bending section

Two separate wires travel from the control lever in the body to the tip of the fibrescope. When the control lever is pressed downwards, the wire that controls the anterior deflection becomes tight and the tip moves anteriorly. The reverse happens when the control lever is moved upwards. The distal bending section houses the tip and is the most flexible section of the fibrescope. In the Olympus LF-2 fibrescope, the bending section has a range of 120° upwards and downwards. The field of view, which is the cone-shaped visual field afforded by this bending section, is 90°. The bending section moves in only one vertical plane. The insertion cord should not be rotated along its long axis, otherwise the angulation wires will cross each other and result in damage.

Universal light cord

The universal cord transmits light from the external light source to the object via the light transmission bundle in the insertion cord. At the light guide connector end, the universal cord incorporates an ETO sterilizing venting cap. This cap should be shut when the fibrescope is sterilized in ethylene oxide, to prevent vacuum from damaging the rubber parts of the insertion cord. The venting cap should also be shut when the fibrescope is being transported. During use and during cleaning and disinfection, the ETO venting cap should be open so that there is no leakage of solution into the insertion cord.

● Light sources, camera and monitor

Light sources

The light guide cable and light source form the bulky part of fibreoptic equipment. Earlier light sources were large, difficult to move and brightness was achieved only at the cost of size. Currently, smaller halogen light sources of 150 W, enclosed in a case weighting just 3 kg, are available. Fibrescopes that can be powered both by an external light source and a battery are also available (e.g. Olympus LF-GP and Pentax FI-10BS). The battery casing replaces the light guide cable and contains a lithium battery that can last for about 60 min (Figure 1.5). A simple flick

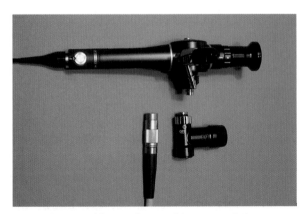

Figure 1.5 Body of a portable intubating fibrescope (Olympus LF-GP). The battery casing and light guide cable are interchangeable

of the battery casing acts as an on–off switch. This arrangement affords versatility and portability to the equipment. It should be possible to move, within a very short time, the fibrescope from one operating theatre to another, to the intensive care unit or to the trauma room where it can be used in an emergency.

Camera and monitor (Figure 1.6)

Use of a camera and monitor facilitates training in fibreoptic endoscopy and intubation. The camera control unit (CCU) is the 'box' to which is connected a camera lead. The other end of the

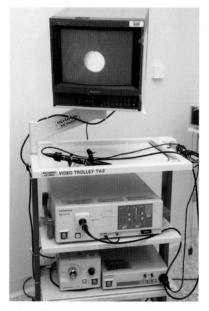

Figure 1.6 An intubating fibrescope connected to a camera control unit which transmits images to a closed circuit television monitor

camera lead has a camera head that is connected to the eyepiece of the fibrescope. The CCU is powered by the fibreoptic light source and receives signals from the camera lead which are then transmitted to a closed circuit television (CCTV) monitor. The size of the image on the CCTV monitor depends on the optical quality and the number of fibres in the image transmission bundle of the fibrescope. For example, the image from an Olympus LF-GP fibrescope with 16 000 fibres is about two and a

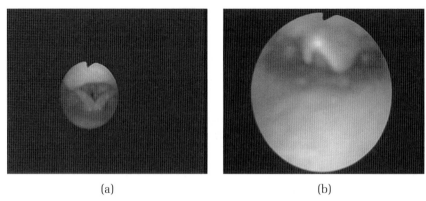

(a)   (b)

Figure 1.7   Comparison of image size from (a) an Olympus LF-2 and (b) an Olympus LF-GP intubating fibrescope

half times bigger than the image from an Olympus LF-2 fibrescope with 6000 fibres (Figure 1.7a,b). A video recorder can be connected to the CCU to record endoscopy pictures.

● Care, cleaning and disinfection of fibreoptic equipment

Care and maintenance

Flexible fibrescopes are expensive equipment and deserve appropriate care. Lenses and fibreoptic bundles are delicate and excessive force or bending will damage them. During use, care must be taken not to force the instrument in the air passage if resistance is encountered. A bite block may be used in the awake patient undergoing oral fibreoptic intubation. All the cables should be off the ground to prevent damage caused by stamping on them. The fibrescope should be hung in a dedicated cupboard so that the insertion cord stays straight (Figure 1.8). The carrying case should only be used for transport. One or two members of the anaesthetic nursing staff or operating department assistants should take responsibility for the general maintenance and a consultant anaesthetist should be in charge overall.

A leakage test should be performed before each session by connecting the venting cap on the light guide cable to a leakage tester. Once the fibrescope is pressurized with air, it is immersed in water and any leaks identified as bubbles. A yearly service check can identify problems early and avoid costly repairs.

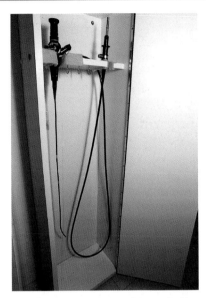

Figure 1.8 The flexible fibrescope is stored in a dedicated cupboard so that the insertion cord stays straight

Cleaning

Staff should wear gloves and eyeglasses to protect them from being splashed with blood, secretions and disinfectant. Cleaning is required to remove the debris and ensure that the optics are clean. Thorough cleaning can also remove 99.9% of the microorganisms and ensures better contact between the disinfectant and remaining microorganisms. Cleaning with tepid soapy water (not Hibiscrub) is satisfactory and should be done immediately after the fibrescope has been used, to prevent blood and secretions drying out.

Disinfection and sterilization

Disinfection reduces microorganisms to a safe level but is not active against bacterial spores and all viruses. **Sterilization** kills all microorganisms including bacterial spores and viruses. Flexible fibreoptic instruments should never be subjected to sterilization at temperatures exceeding 65°C. Ethylene oxide sterilization is satisfactory, but boiling and autoclaving should never be attempted. Chemical disinfection is the usual method; a summary of the properties of some chemical disinfectants is shown in Table 1.1 and a more detailed account follows.

Table 1.1 Properties of commonly used disinfectants

	2% Glutaral-dehyde (Cidex®)	Peracetic acid (PeraSafe®)	Chlorine dioxide (Tristel®)
Disinfection	10 min	5 min	5 min
HIV/mycobacteria	1 h	5 min	10 min
Sterilization	10 h	10 min	10 min
Product life	14/28 days	1 day	14 days
Skin irritant	Yes	No	No
Respiratory irritant	Yes	No	No
Eye irritant	Yes	Yes	No
Corrosive	No	No	No*

*Chlorine dioxide produces a yellowish discoloration of the white indicators on the insertion cord.

2% glutaraldehyde (Cidex®)

This is the most toxic of the commonly used disinfectants but is still widely used. Risks to staff include irritation of the skin, eyes and the respiratory tract. The recommended safe level is 0.2 ppm. Strategies to reduce health hazards include staff awareness and training, wearing protective clothing, and disinfecting in a special area with ventilation and with automated machines where possible. Levels of glutaraldehyde must be monitored and all staff should have pre-employment checks and offered treatment if symptoms occur.

Peracetic acid (PeraSafe®)

This is available as a powder system for rapid and safe sterilization of flexible fibrescopes. The powder is dissolved in water at 35°C to form peracetyl ions, the active agent of peracetic acid. The solution is blue in colour and has a slight acetic odour. The powder is irritant to the skin and the solution to the eyes. It is recommended that gloves and glasses are worn during use, but there is no need for a special area or equipment for disinfection. The powder has a shelf life of 2 years and the solution of 24 h. It does not corrode the fibrescopes.

Chlorine dioxide (Tristel®)

The mixture of a base (sodium chlorite) which is activated by a blend of organic acids releases chlorine dioxide, which is used as a biocidal agent in the water industry. The advantages of chlorine dioxide include shorter times for disinfection and sterilization. It is non-irritant and a special area and equipment for disinfection are not required. It produces a yellowish discoloration of the white indicators on the insertion cord.

Organization of cleaning, disinfection and sterilization of fibrescopes

One of the major obstacles of introducing fibreoptic intubation as a routine practice is the excuse that cleaning and disinfection of fibrescopes takes a long time and delays operating lists. A further argument is that it takes the anaesthetic assistants away from the theatre. This is true for glutaraldehyde sterilization which is done in special areas. The use of agents such as peracetic acid makes it possible to quickly and safely sterilize fibrescopes in the anaesthetic room (Figure 1.9). In our practice, each cycle takes about 15 min.

Advice from the local infection control unit should be sought when a fibreoptic intubation service is planned. It is helpful to explain to them the requirement of a safe, fast and easy system. In our department, the anaesthetic assistants clean and disinfect the fibrescope, but the anaesthetist using the equipment is ultimately responsible. A laminated copy of the cleaning and disinfection

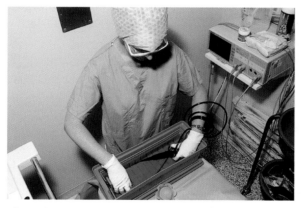

Figure 1.9 Cleaning and disinfection of flexible fibrescopes with peracetic acid (Perasafe®) in the anaesthetic room is convenient

protocol is freely available in the theatre areas and also on the fibreoptic trolley. All trainee anaesthetists are taught how to clean and disinfect fibrescopes in their training module.

Example of a cleaning and disinfection protocol with PeraSafe®

1. The solution is prepared fresh each morning according to the manufacturer's instruction and stored in plastic baths in the anaesthetic room.
2. The fibrescope is cleaned and disinfected at the beginning and end of each operating list and between patients as follows.
3. Flush the working channel with warm water as soon as possible after the fibrescope has been used in a patient.
4. Remove the suction cap and valve, clean the port and working channel with tepid soapy water with the special brushes provided.
5. Immerse the fibrescope, suction cap and valve in the solution and set the stopwatch to alarm at 10 min (Figure 1.10).

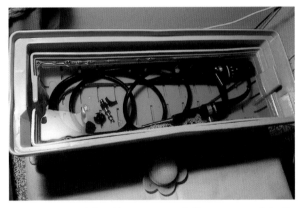

Figure 1.10   The whole of the fibrescope is fully immersed in Perasafe® for 10 min. The suction cap and valve have been removed, cleaned and are also immersed

6. After 10 min, remove the fibrescope from the disinfectant and rinse with sterile water.
7. Flush the working channel with sterile water in a 20 ml syringe.
8. Clean the suction valve and cap in water and replace them.

9. Wipe the outside dry and perform suction through the suction valve to confirm that no fluid remains in the channel.
10. Check the fibrescope (see below) before use in a patient.

● Checking fibreoptic equipment

It is not only important to understand the working principles of fibreoptic equipment, but also to be able to check it before use. Inadequate checks cause faults and are a common source of failure of fibreoptic intubation. As with the anaesthetic machine, every anaesthetist should check fibreoptic equipment before use.

Example of a simple checklist for fibreoptic equipment

1. Ensure that the fibrescope has been cleaned and disinfected before every use.
2. Check the mechanical function by ensuring that the tip moves in the appropriate direction when the control lever is moved and that there is no slack between the control lever and tip motion.
3. Attach a suction catheter to the suction port and ensure that the suction works when the suction valve is activated.
4. Plug the light guide cable to the light source and switch it on.
5. Defog the lens by wiping it with an alcohol swab.
6. Keep the tip of the fibrescope at about 1 cm from an object (usually a letter on a machine) and adjust the dioptre ring so that a clear sharp image appears in the eyepiece.
7. Lubricate the insertion cord (but not the tip), load the tracheal tube on the conical section of the body and secure it with a small piece of tape.

The fibrescope is now ready to use.

The following steps are relevant if a CCU is used with the fibrescope:

1. Check connections between the CCTV and CCU and at the mains and switch on the CCTV.
2. Switch on the CCU and connect it to the fibrescope with the camera cable.
3. Adjust the orientation mark (e.g. 12 o'clock for a supine patient and anaesthetist standing behind the patient) and lock the camera head onto the fibrescope.

4. Adjust the dioptre ring on the camera head for final focusing so that a sharp image is focused on the CCTV monitor.
5. Perform white balance before using the fibrescope and camera on the patient to get the best colour.

The above description is for the most basic CCU and CCTV equipment. The anaesthetist must familiarize himself/herself with the camera equipment by following the manufacturer's instructions.

● Choice of flexible fibrescopes

There is a wide range of intubating fibreoptic equipment available from different manufacturers. Flexible fibrescopes are expensive and careful planning ensures that the right equipment is bought and funds are not wasted. The considerations include the main purpose for which the equipment is bought (theatre use, intensive care or both; or specialist use, e.g. paediatrics) and whether teaching is a priority. The specifications of some of the fibrescopes are shown in Table 1.2. The best fibrescope for theatre use is one of the intubating varieties, e.g. Olympus LF-2 or Pentax FI-10P2. These fibrescopes are ideal for intubating with tracheal tubes 5 mm and larger. At very little extra cost, battery-powered fibrescopes with the same specifications and the additional advantage of portability are available (Olympus LF-GP and Pentax FI-10BS). The small suction channel in the intubating fibrescopes described is their main drawback. An ideal fibrescope for use in the intensive care unit should have better optics with a wide field of view, powerful suction capability and the option of performing biopsies (e.g. Olympus OES 30). Although this fibrescope may be used for tracheal intubation, its daily use for this purpose is not recommended. It is, however, useful when secretion and/or bleeding are causing difficulties (see Chapter 10). In smaller hospitals, or if sufficient funding is not available for separate fibrescopes for theatre and intensive care use, a fibrescope such as an Olympus LF-TP or Pentax FI-13P is ideal (Table 1.2). Instruments for specialist areas such as the ultrathin (e.g. Olympus LF-P or Pentax FI-7P) fibrescope for paediatric use and for placement and checking of double lumen tubes (e.g. Olympus LF-DP or Pentax FI-9BS) are also available.

Where teaching and training is a priority, investment in a camera and monitor will give dividends. Before commitment to

Table 1.2   Specifications and applications of fibrescopes (LF = Olympus, FI = Pentax)

Fibrescope	Insertion cord diameter	Suction channel	Main use	May be used
LF-2	4.0 mm	1.5 mm	Adult intubation	ICU*, DLEBT†
FI-10P2	3.5 mm	1.4 mm	Adult intubation	ICU, DLEBT
LF-GP	4.1 mm	1.5 mm	Adult intubation	ICU, DLEBT
FI-10BS	3.5 mm	1.4 mm	Adult intubation	ICU, DLEBT
LF-TP	5.2 mm	2.6 mm	Adult intubation	ICU
FI-13P	4.2 mm	1.8 mm	Adult intubation	ICU
OES-30	6.0 mm	2.2 mm	ICU	Adult intubation
LF-DP	3.1 mm	1.2 mm	DLEBT	Adult, paediatric intubation
FI-9BS	3.1 mm	1.2 mm	DLEBT	Adult, paediatric intubation
LF-P	2.2 mm	None	Paediatric intubation	
FI-7P	2.4 mm	None	Paediatric intubation	

*ICU = intensive care use.
†DLEBT = Double lumen endobronchial tube placement and checking.

purchase equipment, most distributors are willing to loan equipment for a trial period. This opportunity should be used for decisions among members of the department and also anaesthetic assistants and managers. A service contract will ensure that the equipment is regularly checked and a replacement is available when repairs are needed.

● References

1. Hopkins HH, Kapany NS. A flexible fiberscope, using static scanning. *Nature* 1954; **173**: 39–41.
2. Hirschowitz BI, Curtiss LE, Peters CW, Pollard HM. Demonstration of a new gastroscope, the 'Fiberscope'. *Gastroenterology* 1958; **35**: 50–53.
3. Murphy P. A fiberoptic endoscope used for nasal intubation. *Anaesthesia* 1967; **22**: 489–91.
4. Ikeda S. Flexible bronchofibrescope. *Ann Otol, Rhinol Laryngol* 1970; **79**: 916–23.
5. Taylor PA, Towey RM. The broncho-fibrescope as an aid to endotracheal intubation. *Br J Anaesth* 1972; **44**: 611–12.

6. Conyers AB, Wallace DH, Mulder DS. Use of the fiberoptic bronchoscope for nasotracheal intubation: a case report. *Can Anaesth Soc J* 1972; **19:** 654–6.
7. Stiles CM, Stiles QR, Denson JS. A flexible fiberoptic laryngoscope. *JAMA* 1972; **221:** 1246–7.
8. Davis NJ. A new fiberoptic laryngoscope for nasal intubation. *Anesth Analg* 1973; **52:** 807–8.
9. Prithvi Raj P, Forestner J, Watson TD et al. Techniques for fiberoptic laryngoscopy in anesthesia. *Anesth Analg* 1974; **53(5):** 708–14.

2

Training in fibreoptic intubation

- Introduction
- Oxford fibreoptic training programme
- Pre-clinical module
- Clinical module
- Applications in anaesthesia and intensive care
- Organization of training
- Consent for teaching fibreoptic intubation in anaesthetized patients

● Introduction

Many anaesthetists view using an intubating fibrescope with trepidation. This is because they have not been trained to use a fibrescope properly and often their first case is a patient with a difficult airway who requires an awake fibreoptic intubation. When this results in failure, frustration sets in, the anaesthetist views using a fibrescope as an impossible task and the instrument sits in the cupboard.

Unlike conventional laryngoscopy, which has been taught to most anaesthetists on anaesthetized patients as soon as they start their first jobs, fibreoptic intubation cannot be taught in the time-honoured 'see one, do one' fashion. The fibrescope is a complex intubating tool and requires a degree of skill in using it. Good results are achieved only by learning these skills in a structured and organized way.

The best way is to break the learning process into components and teach/learn each step at a time. This forms the basis of a structured programme. There are many ways in which a structured training programme can be organized [1,2]. The essential rules are that the trainee is given ample opportunity to understand the equipment and practise manual and visual skills on models before being taught on patients. We have developed one such stepwise structured programme for training in fibreoptic endoscopy and intubation in Oxford [3]. The details of this programme are discussed in this chapter.

● Oxford fibreoptic training programme

The details of techniques used for training in the various steps of the programme are the subject of some of the chapters in this book. The steps of the programme are summarized in Table 2.1.

Table 2.1   Oxford fibreoptic training programme

Pre-clinical module
1. Introduction and demonstration of fibreoptic equipment
2. Discussion of the principles of fibreoptic intubation techniques
3. Video demonstration of fibreoptic endoscopy and intubation techniques in anaesthetized and awake patients
4. Practice on the 'Oxford' Fibreoptic Teaching Box and manikins

Clinical module
5. Practise nasal and oral fibreoptic endoscopy and intubation in anaesthetized patients with normal airways
6. Demonstration of upper airway anaesthesia and sedation techniques for awake fibreoptic intubation
7. Practise supervised awake fibreoptic intubation on patients with a difficult airway

The programme has been separated into a pre-clinical and clinical module to emphasize the importance of classroom teaching before training is provided on patients.

● Pre-clinical module

We organize this module in a training room once in every two or three months. Several trainees attend at one time and tuition is provided away from the pressures of the operating theatre. The value of a dedicated room for training in airway skills has been recommended [4].

The objectives of this module are to familiarize the trainee with fibreoptic instruments, including their working principles, setting-up, and cleaning and disinfection procedures (see Chapter 1). Lectures are given on the application of fibreoptic intubation techniques in anaesthetized and awake patients. The reader will find information on these in the appropriate chapters in this book. In the third step of this module, trainees are shown video recordings of some of these techniques. The topics include demonstration of both good and bad fibreoptic endoscopy techniques, methods of topical anaesthesia of the upper airway and techniques of awake fibreoptic intubation. Videos form an excellent medium of instruction. It is easy to connect a video recorder to the endoscopic camera during fibreoptic procedures and obtain a good collection of videos for use in classroom teaching.

The final and most important step in this module is to give trainees ample opportunity to practise on models and manikins to learn and gain confidence in fibreoptic manipulation skills. Many models are available for training. We have developed our own, the 'Oxford' Fibreoptic Teaching Box (see Chapter 3). This practice is essential in developing hand–eye coordination and visual skills. Practice is also provided on manikins for the learning principles of railroading tracheal tubes. Trainees are encouraged to practise both with and without a camera and monitor system in order to familiarize themselves with endoscopy appearances on both the monitor and the eyepiece.

At the end of this module, trainees are well prepared for their first encounter with fibreoptic techniques on a patient. We consider this pre-clinical module an essential part of our training programme and insist that trainees complete it before they proceed to supervised training on patients.

● Clinical module

The ultimate objective of our structured programme is for the trainee to perform safe and successful fibreoptic intubation on patients. Opportunity is provided in the first step of this module to consolidate manipulation skills on anaesthetized patients. Emphasis is placed on mastering meticulous endoscopy techniques in order to guide the tip of the fibrescope toward the laryngeal inlet in an unhurried and atraumatic fashion. The trainees learn to keep the tip of the fibrescope in the middle of the visual field by appropriate manipulation. They begin to appreciate the problems of secretions, blood and of airway collapse, among many other things, and learn how to manage them. It is uncertain how many fibreoptic intubations trainees need to perform in anaesthetized patients before they can be deemed competent. We continuously assess each trainee and feel that some learn fast and others take longer. Some of the techniques we use for teaching fibreoptic endoscopy and intubation in anaesthetized patients are discussed in Chapter 6.

The final two stages of this module involve teaching awake fibreoptic intubation techniques. It is vital that trainees' endoscopy skills are immaculate before practising on awake patients. They are first shown how to provide 'conscious' sedation (see Chapter 8) and perform local anaesthesia of the upper airway (see Chapter 9) for awake fibreoptic intubation. Finally they are allowed to perform awake fibreoptic intubation under supervision. This is the most difficult part of the programme. We have achieved reasonable teaching of awake intubation by targeting a maxillofacial list where a high proportion of patients need awake intubation. As the trainers and the whole theatre team have gained confidence in the programme, the threshold for awake intubation has decreased, making the availability of suitable cases for teaching much easier.

● Applications in anaesthesia and intensive care

The primary goal of our structured programme is to provide training for achieving competency in performing fibreoptic intubation. Some more applications of fibrescopes include diagnostic bronchoscopy in intensive care, placement and positioning check of double lumen tubes, changing tracheal tubes and during percutaneous tracheostomy (see Chapter 12). Although these are not formally taught in our programme, every opportunity is taken to demonstrate and teach these techniques to trainees.

● Organization of training

The problems of training in fibreoptic intubation and some of their solutions have been reviewed [5,6]. There is no doubt about the value of a structured programme such as the one mentioned.

The problems are of putting the principles of the programme into clinical practice. Achieving this goal is a matter of teamwork and the role of some important factors is considered.

Trainers

Consultants who aspire to become trainers in fibreoptic intubation should be knowledgeable, experienced and routinely performing these techniques in their clinical practice. Not all consultants in a department would be able to fulfil this role and the best way is for a small group to organize the training. It is likely that many new consultants would have had training and experience as trainees themselves and they should be able to set up training programmes in their own departments. For others, it may be worth attending one of the several practical workshops. Informal visits to departments where fibreoptic techniques are practised routinely are very helpful. Trainers should be committed to teaching in the classroom and in the theatre.

Equipment

The need for an airway training room has already been emphasized in teaching the pre-clinical module. The value of fibreoptic equipment with a camera and monitor for training has been established [2]. Ancillary equipment for use in theatre and in the classroom should also be available.

Cleaning and disinfection

One of the major obstacles to fibreoptic intubation training is the need to clean and sterilize instruments between each case. This is usually given as a reason for delaying surgical lists and for not teaching fibreoptic intubation. A simple and effective method of sterilizing fibreoptic equipment with peracetic acid in the anaesthetic room will avoid these problems (see Chapter 1).

Training lists

The number of intubations performed for elective surgery has dramatically decreased in recent years. This is partly due to the use of other airway devices, namely the laryngeal mask airway and the use of regional techniques. It is therefore important to target those operating lists for fibreoptic training where intubation is still routinely performed. Oral surgery lists are ideal for teaching nasotracheal intubation, but others, for example general surgical or gynaecological lists, can also effectively be used.

Anaesthetic assistants

Anaesthetic assistants are important members of the training team. Discussions should always take place about the impact of training on their workload and cooperation sought from the beginning. They have an important role when fibreoptic techniques are taught (see Chapters 6 and 9).

Surgeons

Surgeons and many anaesthetists have a misconception that fibreoptic training delays lists and slows patient turnover. This is not always true if proper planning is in place. The cooperation of surgeons should be sought before setting up teaching lists.

Education

Education is important in disseminating newer ideas. As with the introduction of any new technique in anaesthesia, it is important to educate all medical and nursing staff involved. It is a satisfying experience to see the reward of one's hard work in setting up a training programme. The reward is well-trained young anaesthetists who would be consultants of the future.

● Consent for teaching fibreoptic intubation in anaesthetized patients

Some anaesthetists are concerned about the ethics of teaching fibreoptic intubation in anaesthetized patients. In the UK, the Association of Anaesthetists' document *Information and Consent for Anaesthesia* [7] recommends at least verbal consent for anaesthesia, but suggests that it is unnecessary to detail each individual anaesthetic procedure to the patient if it is routinely performed. It further states that trying to get consent for each individual procedure may lead to restricted consent, i.e. the patient may agree to have a general anaesthetic but refuse intubation.

The question is whether fibreoptic intubation under general anaesthesia causes additional risks to the patient and whether it should be considered a routine procedure. Many studies have compared fibreoptic intubation with conventional intubation and confirmed that it is safe for both orotracheal and nasotracheal intubation (see Chapter 6).

Trainers in fibreoptic intubation must have the necessary experience to consider fibreoptic intubation as a **routine** procedure in their clinical practice before teaching others. Airway experts on both sides of the Atlantic have debated the need for a specific patient consent for teaching airway techniques, particularly fibreoptic intubation. In the USA, Benumof does not consider this necessary in his training programme [8]. In the UK, the majority of anaesthetists at a Difficult Airway Society debate voted that teaching airway management on unconsented patients is not unethical [9].

At the present time, there is lack of standard guidelines for training in fibreoptic intubation. A trainer is advised to seek local guidance before embarking on training fibreoptic intubation in anaesthetized patients with normal airway.

• References

1. Ovassapian A, Dykes MHM, Golman ME. A training programme for fibreoptic nasotracheal intubation. Use of model and live patients. *Anaesthesia* 1983; **38:** 795–8.
2. Smith JE, Fenner SG, King MJ. Teaching fibreoptic nasotracheal intubation with and without closed circuit television. *Br J Anaesth* 1993; **71:** 206–11.
3. Popat MT. Teaching and training in fibreoptic intubation. *CPD Anaesthesia* 2000; **2:** 66–71.
4. Mason RA. Education and training in airway management. *Br J Anaesth* 1998; **81:** 305–7.
5. Mason RA. Learning fibreoptic intubation: fundamental problems. *Anaesthesia* 1992; **47:** 729–31.
6. Vaughan RS. Training in fibreoptic laryngoscopy. *Br J Anaesth* 1991; **66:** 538–40.
7. Association of Anaesthetists of Great Britain and Ireland. *Information and Consent for Anaesthesia*, pp. 3–5. London, 1999.
8. Benumof JL, Cooper SD. Teaching airway management skills: What about patient consent? *Anaesthesiology* 1996; **85:** 438–9.
9. Popat M. Teaching airway management on unconsented patients is unethical (against). *Difficult Airway Society Abstracts*, Edinburgh 1999; 26–7.

3

Learning basic fibreoptic endoscopy skills

● Manipulations of flexible intubating fibrescopes

Holding the fibrescope

The endoscopist holds the body of the fibrescope in the palm of one hand (left or right) and the insertion cord with the thumb and index finger of the other hand. The thumb of the hand that holds the body manipulates the control lever and its index finger activates the suction channel when required (Figure 3.1a). The insertion cord is held straight and taut at all times (Figure 3.1b). If the insertion cord is allowed to bow or become slack, rotation movements of the body will not be effectively transmitted to the tip of the fibrescope.

Manipulating the tip of the fibrescope

There are three ways in which an endoscopist can manipulate the tip of the fibrescope towards the desired target. These are advancement (or withdrawal), tip deflection and rotation. Advancing the whole fibrescope moves it towards the target. Sometimes withdrawal is required if the fibrescope has been advanced too far. The control lever on the body moves the tip of the fibrescope in a vertical plane (anteriorly or posteriorly) only. When the control lever is pressed down, the tip bends anteriorly (or away from the endoscopist); when the control lever is moved

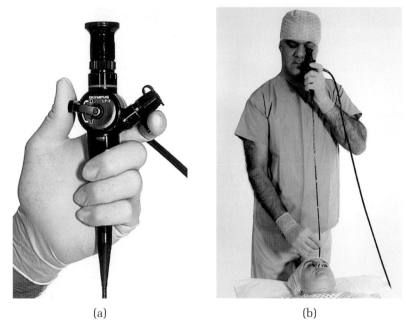

(a)   (b)

Figure 3.1   (a) The body of the fibrescope is held in the palm of one hand. The thumb manipulates the control lever and the index finger activates the suction channel; (b) the insertion cord of the fibrescope is held straight and taut at all times

up, the tip faces posteriorly (or towards the endscopist). The sideways movements of the tip are achieved by rotation of the body of the fibrescope towards the target while maintaining tip deflection. In practice, a good endoscopy technique involves performing the three basic manipulations simultaneously in order to bring the tip of the fibrescope towards the target. When viewed in the eyepiece or on the monitor, an orientation marker indicates the anterior direction of tip movement.

These concepts are illustrated in a simplified diagram (Figure 3.2). The visual field, through an eyepiece or on a monitor screen, is represented by a circle with four quadrants. The orientation marker is at the 12 o'clock position. Imagine that the tip of the fibrescope is in a neutral position in the centre of the field at the point O and has to be moved to a point A. This is facilitated by deflecting the tip anteriorly and at the same time rotating the body in a clockwise direction. Similarly, a posterior tip deflection and anticlockwise rotation will bring the tip from

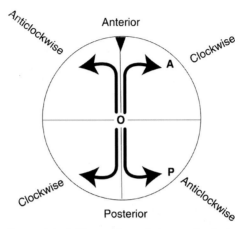

Figure 3.2   Two-dimensional illustration of tip manipulation. The visual field is represented by a circle with four quadrants. Tip deflection and rotation of body are required to move the tip of the fibrescope from O to A or P. See text for details

the point O to the target P. In reality the process is three dimensional and advancement of the fibrescope is needed with other movements.

Position of the endoscopist and patient

The anaesthetist should be comfortable when performing fibreoptic endoscopy. A platform must be used instead of standing on tiptoe and trying to get enough height to keep the insertion cord straight. If this is not done, fatigue of the arms will rapidly ensue and inevitably the insertion cord will slacken and bow. Another way of holding is to angle the body of the fibrescope, towards the endoscopist, at its junction with the insertion cord. The effective length of the fibrescope is reduced, but the insertion cord remains taut and the operator is comfortable. A common problem is of the operator moving his/her own body rather than the body of the fibrescope! Although entertaining to onlookers, this should be avoided.

The operator may choose to stand behind the head, in front of or on either side of the patient facing them. The patient may be supine or lying on the side. Some anaesthetists prefer to perform awake intubation with the patient sitting. In the beginning of their training, we prefer that trainees learn to recognize the anatomy of the upper airway on the monitor screen while standing behind a supine patient's head. Anaesthetists are most familiar with this position and the airway anatomy is similar to that seen during conventional direct laryngoscopy. With practice and confidence, the appearances of the visual fields in other positions can also be learnt.

● Learning manual dexterity and hand–eye coordination on models

During fibreoptic endoscopy the 'eye' is at the objective lens in the tip of the fibrescope, unlike direct laryngoscopy, where the movement of the laryngoscope handle and blade are observed with the naked eye. Hence, mastering fibreoptic skills requires not only a thorough understanding of the working principles of the instrument, but a lot of practice in manipulation skills. Initial practice is best gained on teaching models. Several types of model are available, but the main objective is to give the trainee a chance to understand how the different manipulations at the body of the fibrescope are translated to the tip. An indication of achieving perfect manual dexterity and hand–eye coordination is a state when one is not consciously thinking of the manipulations while performing them. The mind does the job. It is like learning to drive a car where initially one has to think each time before changing gear, but after practice the hands do this without the mind telling them. It is important to master these manipulation skills thoroughly on teaching boxes and models before practising on patients. The common models used for teaching fibreoptic manipulation skills are the Laerdal® bronchial tree model [1], and various 'hit the hole' boxes [2–4]. We have developed one, the 'Oxford' Fibreoptic Teaching Box, a short description of which follows.

● The 'Oxford' Fibreoptic Teaching Box (Figure 3.3a)

The box has four rectangular sides with a square top and bottom and measures 40 cm × 20 cm × 20 cm. Up to eight square plates can be slid into or removed from the box by lifting one of the rectangular sides. The plates have holes, each of about 6 mm diameter, drilled into them. All the plates have a different arrangement of holes surrounding one central hole. The distance between any two plates is approximately 5 cm. The size and arrangement of the holes in the box is selected so that the tip of an adult intubating fibrescope (Olympus LF-2) just passes through them only when actively manipulated. The holes have chamfered edges to prevent damage to the fibrescope. By practising on the box, trainees get a spatial orientation of fibrescope manipulation with a combination of advancement, rotation and tip deflection. Most importantly, they appreciate

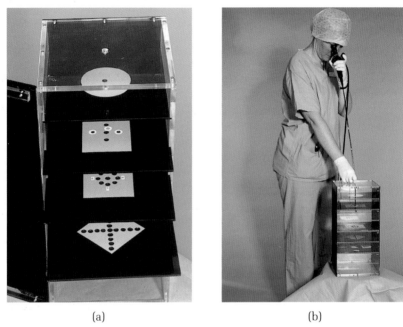

(a)   (b)

Figure 3.3   The 'Oxford' Fibreoptic Teaching Box: (a) one of the sides is lifted open to demonstrate the arrangements of plates and holes; (b) trainee practising manipulation skills in the anaesthetic room

that only subtle movements are required and that keeping the tip of the fibrescope in the centre of the visual field with a combination of manipulations achieves the highest success.

The usefulness of this teaching box has been confirmed in a randomized controlled trial [5]. When assessed on an intubating manikin, trainees who had practice on the box showed significantly better manipulation skills than trainees who had not. The advantages of this box are its simple design, low manufacturing cost and virtually no maintenance. It is lightweight and portable. We keep one in an anaesthetic room so that trainees can practise manipulation skills whenever they find an opportunity (Figure 3.3b).

Practice on intubating manikins

Most basic intubating manikins are designed for teaching direct laryngoscopy skills, since the airway anatomy is nothing like it is in a real patient. Advanced manikins are expensive. Once the trainees have gained manual dexterity skills on the teaching box, practice on the manikins is useful for learning the appearance of the visual fields during nasal and oral endoscopy. The manikin can be placed in different positions (supine, side or sitting) and the trainee can practise fibreoptic endoscopy by standing behind the head, on the side or in front. Another use of the manikin is for demonstration of the principles of tracheal tube selection and railroading techniques.

References

1. Smith JE, Jackson APF, Hurdley J, Clifton PJM. Learning curves for fibreoptic nasotracheal intubation when using the endoscopic video camera. *Anaesthesia* 1997; **52:** 101–6.
2. Bainton CR. Models to facilitate the learning of fiberoptic technique. In: Bainton CR, ed. *New Concepts in Airway Management. International Anesthesiology Clinics.* Boston, Little Brown 1994; **32:** 47–55.
3. Nott MR. A trainer for fibreoptic intubation. *Anaesthesia* 1995; **50:** 570–71.
4. Williams KA, Harwood RJ, Woodall NM, Barker GL. Training in fibreoptic intubation. *Anaesthesia* 2000; **55:** 99–100.
5. Popat M, Benham SW, Kapila A, Addy V. Randomised controlled trial of learning fibreoptic skills on the 'Oxford' training box. *Difficult Airway Society Abstracts*, Edinburgh 1999; 61–2.

4

Airway aids for fibreoptic intubation

Mansukh Popat and Atul Kapila

- Definition of fibreoptic airway aids
- Conduit airways
- Ventilation aids
- Combined conduit and ventilation aids
- LMA-assisted orotracheal fibreoptic intubation
- LMA-assisted nasotracheal fibreoptic intubation

● Definition of fibreoptic airway aids

It is not always possible (or desirable) to perform fibreoptic intubation by simply guiding the tip of the fibrescope into the trachea and railroading a tracheal tube over it. Some form of airway device may be required to facilitate insertion of the fibrescope and/or maintain ventilation of the patient. These devices are collectively referred to as 'fibreoptic airway aids' in this book. Many such aids have been described; examples of some of the more commonly used fibreoptic aids are shown in Table 4.1.

● Conduit airways

These special airways are useful for fibreoptic intubation by the orotracheal route. The oropharynx has a large airspace, and it is difficult to keep the tip of the fibrescope in the midline. When inserted in the oropharynx, these airways will lift the tongue from the posterior pharyngeal wall and create a conduit for the tip of the fibrescope. They help to keep the tip of the fibrescope in the midline and guide it to the larynx. They can

Table 4.1 Fibreoptic airway aids

Conduit airways
Ovassapian Airway
Berman II Airway
Bronchoscope Airway (VBM®)
Williams Airway Intubator

Ventilation aids
Patil–Syracuse Mask
Endoscopy Mask (VBM®)
Modified facemask
Chimney airway
Cuffed nasopharyngeal airway

Combined conduit and ventilation aids
Laryngeal mask airway
Intubating laryngeal mask airway
Cuffed oropharyngeal airway

be used for fibreoptic intubation in the anaesthetized or awake patient, when they will also prevent damage to the fibrescope by patients biting on it. These airways are not designed to deliver anaesthetic gases or oxygen to the patient. In its simplest form, an ordinary Guedel airway slit longitudinally will serve the purpose, but the following airways are specifically designed.

Ovassapian Airway (Figure 4.1)

This airway was designed by Professor Andranik Ovassapian of Chicago, USA [1]. A disposable airway, it has a narrow squared proximal portion which acts as a bite block and a broad curved distal lingual portion which presses against the tongue and prevents it from falling back and obstructing the airspace. An intubating fibrescope with or without a tracheal tube of size 8 mm and smaller can easily be passed through this airway. Once intubation is complete, the airway can be peeled back and removed from the mouth. Its main disadvantage is that it is available in only one size.

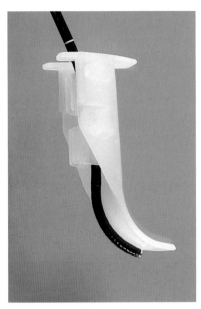

Figure 4.1 Ovassapian Airway, showing position of an intubating fibrescope through its lumen

Berman II Airway (Figure 4.2)

This airway has been successfully used for orotracheal fibreoptic intubation [2], although it was originally designed for assisting oral blind intubation [3]. It is tubular in shape, available in four sizes and is disposable. When properly inserted it will keep the tip of the fibrescope in the midline and guide it to the larynx. The airway has a plastic hinge down the left side and a lateral opening down the right side from where it can be peeled open and removed. When this airway was compared with the tongue traction method for assisting orotracheal intubation, no differences in intubation times were found [2].

Bronchoscope Airway (VBM®) (Figure 4.3)

This disposable oropharyngeal airway is available in four sizes. The cross-section of the proximal half of the airway is 'C' shaped, acting as a conduit for the fibrescope and allowing its tip to stay in the midline. The distal lingual surface is flat and prevents the tongue from falling onto the posterior pharyngeal wall and obstructing the airspace. The bite block portion is padded, giving

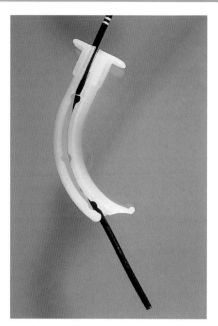

Figure 4.2 Berman II Airway, showing position of an intubating fibrescope through its lumen

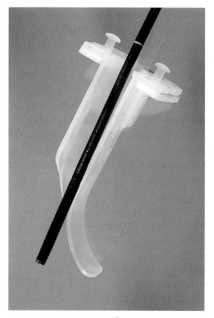

Figure 4.3 Bronchoscope airway (VBM®), showing position of an intubating fibrescope through its lumen

protection to the fibrescope and lips from an accidental bite. A side channel on the left allows suctioning of the oropharynx during fibreoptic endoscopy if required. The steps for using these airways for oropharyngeal fibreoptic intubation in anaesthetized patients are described in Chapter 6.

● Ventilation aids

It is vitally important to maintain oxygenation and keep the patient anaesthetized while fibreoptic endoscopy and intubation are taking place. The following ventilation aids can generally help with this function, but they do not act as conduits for the fibrescope. Their use has declined since the introduction of airway aids that act both as conduits and ventilation devices, described later in this chapter.

Patil–Syracuse Mask [4]

This rubber facemask has a separate port for insertion of the fibrescope while anaesthesia is maintained with the breathing system connected to the normal port. A rubber diaphragm covering the dedicated port prevents leakage of anaesthetic gases when the fibrescope is inserted into the mask. Problems have been reported with the rubber diaphragm tearing and being pushed into the trachea during railroading. The rubber diaphragm is also expensive to replace.

Endoscopy Mask (VBM®)

This mask is clear, disposable and available in three sizes (neonates, children and adults). The removable silicone diaphragm on top of the mask has a small hole that allows insertion of the tip of the fibrescope without leakage of anaesthetic gases (Figure 4.4a). When endoscopy is complete, the tracheal tube is advanced through this hole which expands and allows the tube to enter through it (Figure 4.4b). The mask can be removed from the silicone diaphragm, leaving it attached to the tracheal tube for later removal (Figure 4.4c). The mask has a separate port to which the breathing system is connected.

Modified facemask

An ordinary facemask can be modified to assist fibreoptic intubation when no specific equipment is available (Figure 4.5).

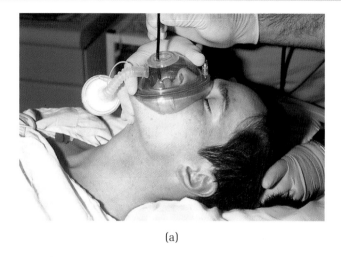

(a)

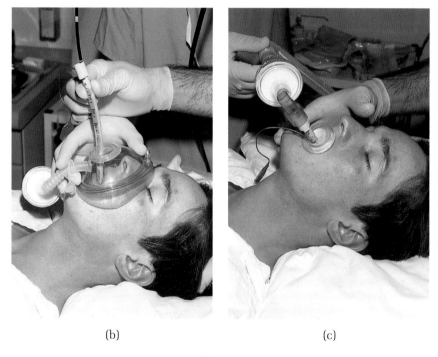

(b)   (c)

Figure 4.4 Endoscopy mask (VBM®). The removable silicone diaphragm
has a hole which allows insertion of the fibrescope through it. The mask has
a separate port to which the breathing system is attached (a). The tracheal
tube is advanced through the hole in the diaphragm (b). The mask is
removed but the silicone diaphragm stays attached to the tube (c)

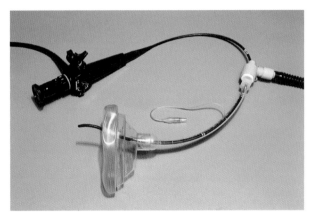

Figure 4.5 A facemask/tracheal tube assembly for assisting fibreoptic intubation. See text for details

The angle piece of the mask is removed, and a tracheal tube is passed through the mask such that its inflated cuff will keep the tube in the mask and provide an airtight seal [5]. The 15 mm connector of the tracheal tube is attached to the breathing system via a swivel diaphragm connector and fibreoptic endoscopy performed via the tracheal tube. When the tip of the fibrescope is in the trachea, railroading of the tracheal tube is completed after the cuff has been deflated. The 15 mm connector is disconnected to allow removal of the mask.

The masks described above can be used for orotracheal or nasotracheal fibreoptic intubation. When used for orotracheal intubation, a conduit airway may be used to guide the fibrescope to the larynx. They can also be used both in spontaneously breathing or paralysed patients. One disadvantage is that a second pair of hands is required to maintain the airway and position of the mask while the anaesthetist is performing the fibreoptic intubation.

Chimney airway

This is essentially a Guedel airway modified by attaching a 15 mm tracheal tube connector to its proximal end, to allow direct connection to a breathing system (Figure 4.6a). Once it has been inserted, nasotracheal fibreoptic endoscopy and intubation can be achieved while the patient is breathing spontaneously through the airway (Figure 4.6b). Tight strapping with

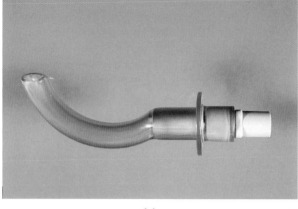

(a)

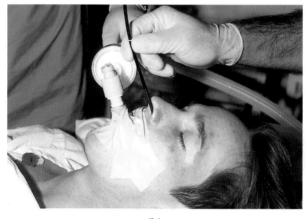

(b)

Figure 4.6 (a) Chimney airway. (b) Nasotracheal endoscopy is carried out while the patient is breathing through the airway. Airtight seal with tape prevents leakage of anaesthetic gases

tape around the mouth will prevent leakage of anaesthetic gas [6].

Cuffed nasopharyngeal airway (CNPA)

This device is a nasopharyngeal airway with a cuff which when inflated sits in the oropharynx, providing a sealed airway and hands-free operation. It can be used in anaesthetized or awake patients. Its main advantage is that it will provide anaesthesia and ventilation via one nostril and permit fibreoptic endoscopy and intubation through the other nostril [7]. It is available in one size of 6 mm internal diameter (ID) and can be used in adult patients only. The CNPA may be useful when mouth opening is limited and a laryngeal mask airway cannot be inserted.

● Combined conduit and ventilation aids

These airway aids can act **both** as a conduit for the fibrescope during orotracheal fibreoptic intubation and as an airway to maintain anaesthesia and ventilation (spontaneous or controlled) during the procedure. This allows fibreoptic intubation to be accomplished in an unhurried and controlled fashion, making the procedure safe for the patient.

Laryngeal mask airway (LMA)

The LMA is the most common airway device currently used in anaesthetic practice. Blind tracheal intubation through the LMA is possible, but the success rate varies between 30% and 97% [8–10]. It can cause trauma to the upper airway and its use cannot be recommended. The advantages of using a LMA as an airway aid for assisting fibreoptic intubation are shown in Table 4.2.

Table 4.2 Advantages of a laryngeal mask airway as a fibreoptic aid

Anaesthetists are familiar with its use
Applicable to all age groups
Can be used in awake or anaesthetized patients
Can be used in spontaneously breathing or paralysed patients
Provides hands-free airway maintenance
Conduit for the fibrescope during orotracheal fibreoptic
    intubation
Can maintain ventilation even in patients with a difficult airway
Recommended for the failed intubation and in the 'can't
    intubate, can't ventilate' scenario

Clinical applications of LMA-assisted fibreoptic intubation

1. Anticipated difficult airway in uncooperative patient not suitable for awake intubation.
2. Unanticipated difficult intubation where rescue ventilation has been possible with a LMA ('can't intubate, can ventilate').
3. 'Can't ventilate, can't intubate', where rescue ventilation has been possible with a LMA [11].
4. Facilitating awake fibreoptic intubation [12].
5. Training in nasotracheal fibreoptic intubation in anaesthetized patients to reduce apnoea time [13].

The success rate of LMA-assisted fibreoptic intubation in the above clinical applications is unknown. This is a common problem in studies involving any airway device because of the number of patients involved. It is true, however, that there is a definite learning curve and teaching LMA-assisted fibreoptic intubation techniques should be part of any fibreoptic training programme.

● LMA-assisted orotracheal fibreoptic intubation
(Table 4.3)

Direct techniques

Standard LMA

A fibrescope (loaded with a tracheal tube) is passed into the lumen of a LMA and guided through its bars into the larynx and

---

Table 4.3   Techniques of LMA-assisted fibreoptic intubation

Orotracheal intubation
Direct techniques
Standard LMA
Modified LMA

Two-stage technique
Aintree Intubation Catheter
Gum elastic bougie
Guide wire

Nasotracheal intubation

trachea. The tracheal tube is then railroaded over the fibrescope with the LMA still in situ. The LMA acts as a conduit for the fibrescope and maintains ventilation during the procedure. The LMA may be left *in situ* after intubation or removed.

Practical steps of direct fibreoptic-assisted intubation through standard LMA

1. Insert a LMA in the usual fashion and confirm ventilation through it.
2. Connect a breathing system to it via a self-sealing swivel connector (Figure 4.7a).

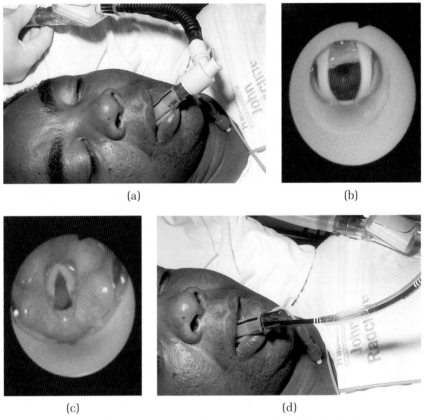

(a) (b)

(c) (d)

Figure 4.7 Direct fibreoptic-assisted intubation through a LMA. Connect a breathing system to the LMA (a). Negotiate the tip of an intubating fibrescope through the bars of the LMA (b) and into the larynx (c). Railroad a tracheal tube over the fibrescope and through the LMA (d)

3. Negotiate the tip of a fibrescope, loaded with a 6 mm tracheal tube, through the bars of the LMA and into the trachea under direct vision until the carina is seen (Figure 4.7b,c).
4. Railroad the tracheal tube over the fibrescope (Figure 4.7d).
5. Confirm the position of the tube with the fibrescope.
6. The LMA can be left in place with the tube secured to it.

Limitations of direct technique using standard LMA

1. It may be difficult to negotiate the tip of the fibrescope through the bars of the LMA because the larynx is usually pushed forwards when the cuff of the LMA is inflated and is angled away from the axial alignment of the pharynx. The fibrescope tip has to negotiate an S-bend by directing it to the epiglottis and then turning sharply into the trachea [14].
2. Tracheal tubes larger than 6 mm ID cannot pass through a size 4 LMA (and 7 mm tracheal tubes through a size 5 LMA).
3. The cuff of the tracheal tube may come to lie within the laryngeal vestibule, even with the tracheal tube fully inserted through the LMA, risking vocal cord damage. This is because the total length of the commonly used uncut cuffed tracheal tubes (e.g. Portex or Mallinkrodt) is about 27 cm. The LMA has a 19 cm long stem. As it has been shown that the average distance between the grille of the LMA and the vocal cords is 3.6 cm in males and 3.1 cm in females [15], only about 4.5 cm of the distal end of the tracheal tube (which includes the cuff) is available for tracheal intubation (Figure 4.8). This problem may be avoided by selecting a longer tracheal tube, e.g. a Mallinkrodt flexometallic which is 33 cm long [16], by using a modified LMA or a two-stage technique (see below). When contemplating this technique, the length of the tracheal tube in relation to the LMA should always be checked.
4. The LMA can be difficult to remove once intubation has been accomplished. The tracheal tube may be left *in situ* if its presence will not interfere with surgical access. When it is necessary to remove the LMA, first the 15 mm connector of the tracheal tube is removed, then the length of the tube is effectively increased by a gum elastic bougie, a tracheal tube changer or a second smaller tube passed through the first tube [17] and the LMA removed.

There is a learning curve for this technique and it should be taught and practised before its use in difficult airway patients.

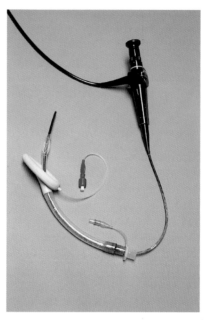

Figure 4.8 Limitation of direct fibreoptic-assisted intubation through a LMA. With the tracheal tube fully inserted, only about 4.5 cm of its distal end (which includes the cuff) is available for tracheal intubation. This makes it possible for the cuff of the tracheal tube to lie in the laryngeal vestibule, risking vocal cord damage

Its reported success rate in patients with a normal airway is 90−97% [18,19].

Modified LMA technique

Some of the limitations of the LMA-assisted fibreoptic intubation using a standard LMA can be overcome by using a modified LMA. Examples include a LMA with a short stem (available in only size 3) or splitting the standard LMA longitudinally and resealing the cuff with vulcanizing silicone. This arrangement allows removal of the LMA after intubation and compared favourably with the Berman II intubating airway as a conduit [20]. The device is not available commercially.

Two-stage techniques

Some of the difficulties with the direct technique can be overcome with a two-stage technique. Instead of directly rail-

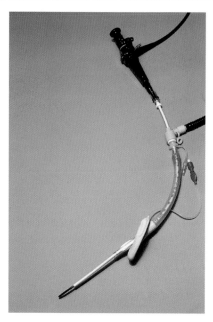

Figure 4.9   The Aintree Intubation Catheter is designed to snugly fit over the insertion cord of an adult intubating fibrescope. It is then railroaded through a LMA into the trachea under direct vision

roading a tracheal tube over the fibrescope, a device such as an Aintree Intubation Catheter, a gum elastic bougie or a guide wire is inserted into the trachea under fibreoptic guidance and the LMA removed (first stage). The tracheal tube is then railroaded over this device (second stage).

Aintree Intubation Catheter technique (Figure 4.9)

The Aintree Intubation Catheter (AIC) was developed in Liverpool and first described in 1996 [21]. It is a sleeve (hollow bougie), 56 cm long and designed to fit snugly over an adult intubating fibrescope (e.g. Olympus LF–2, 4 mm). It was specifically designed for intubation through the LMA. Its flexibility allows loading over the fibrescope and its stiffness facilitates railroading of a tracheal tube.

The steps of using an AIC for a LMA-assisted orotracheal fibreoptic intubation are as follows:

1. Insert a LMA in the usual fashion and confirm ventilation through it by connecting it to a breathing system using a 15 mm fibreoptic swivel connector (Figure 4.10a).

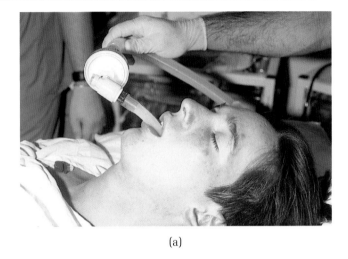

(a)

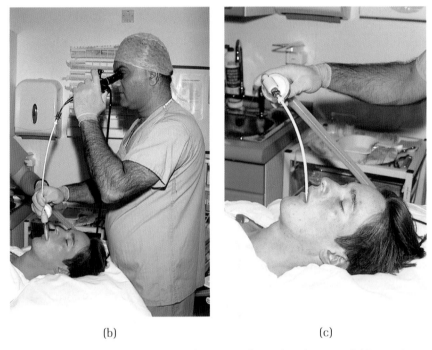

(b)   (c)

Figure 4.10 Steps of Aintree Intubation Catheter (AIC) assisted fibreoptic intubation through LMA. Insert the LMA and connect it to a breathing system via a fibreoptic swivel connector (a). Guide an intubating fibrescope loaded with the AIC through the LMA and into the trachea (b). Remove the LMA and fibrescope (c).

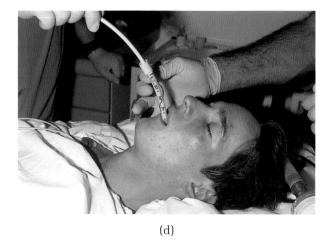

(d)

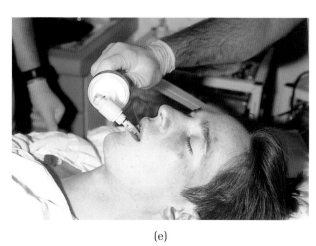

(e)

Figure 4.10 (*continued*)   Railroad a suitable tracheal tube over the AIC (d). Remove the AIC and connect the tracheal tube to the breathing system and check its position (e)

2. Guide an intubating fibrescope loaded with an AIC through the LMA bars and assess the position of the LMA (Figure 4.10b).
3. Advance the fibrescope tip through the larynx and into the trachea.
4. Remove the fibrescope and the LMA leaving the AIC positioned in the trachea (Figure 4.10c).
5. Railroad a suitable size tracheal tube over the AIC (Figure 4.10d).

6. Remove the AIC and check the position of the tracheal tube with end tidal carbon dioxide (Figure 4.10e).

Advantages of the AIC catheter technique

1. LMA can be safely removed.
2. The AIC can maintain ventilation and oxygenation through a standard 15 mm or jet ventilator connector [14].
3. Tracheal tubes larger than 6 mm can be safely used.

This technique is safer, easier and preferred to the direct technique but takes slightly longer.

Gum elastic bougie technique

A gum elastic bougie may be passed blindly through a LMA and negotiated into the glottis. This approach has a high failure rate, and may cause trauma, oedema and bleeding in the larynx. A safer fibreoptic-assisted technique has been described [22], with an 88% success rate.

The steps of the technique are as follows:

1. Insert a LMA in the usual fashion and confirm ventilation through it.
2. Guide an intubating fibrescope through the LMA and negotiate its tip through the bars to lie near the glottis.
3. Pass a gum elastic bougie alongside the fibrescope and negotiate it through the vocal cords under fibreoptic guidance.
4. Remove the fibrescope and LMA and leave the bougie in the trachea.
5. Railroad an appropriate sized tracheal tube over the bougie which is then removed.
6. Confirm the position of the tracheal tube with end tidal carbon dioxide.

This technique is useful when an AIC is unavailable. There is a risk that the bougie may accidentally come out of the trachea when the LMA is removed.

Guide wire technique

This is a useful technique in children (see Chapter 11) and has also been described in adults [23]. The steps of the technique are as follows:

1. Insert a LMA in the usual fashion and confirm ventilation through it.
2. Pass a long guide wire (e.g. Cook retrograde wire – J tip, 0.98 mm thick, 110 cm long or a cardiac catheter wire) through the working channel of the fibrescope.
3. Introduce the fibrescope through LMA and negotiate its tip through the bars and into the trachea.
4. Feed the wire so that a sufficient length is in the trachea.
5. Remove the fibrescope.
6. Pass a small exchange catheter or wire stiffener over the wire.
7. Remove the wire.
8. Railroad a suitable sized tracheal tube over the exchange catheter.

This technique is satisfactory when an AIC is unavailable and is preferred to the bougie technique.

● LMA-assisted nasotracheal fibreoptic intubation

A LMA can provide adequate ventilation and/or anaesthesia during fibreoptic endoscopy and intubation via the nasal route. This technique is useful during training in nasotracheal fibreoptic endoscopy and intubation [13]. The total apnoea time during nasotracheal endoscopy is reduced when a LMA is used as a ventilatory aid in anaesthetized, paralysed patients. Ventilation is continued through the LMA while the trainee performs nasendoscopy. It is then removed and the trainee continues with pharyngoscopy, laryngoscopy and tracheoscopy (see Chapter 6). This technique may also be used in patients with a difficult airway in whom a nasal tube is required. A similar technique has also been described in spontaneously breathing patients anaesthetized with oxygen and halothane [24].

Intubating LMA (ILMA)

This device, introduced by Dr A.I.J. Brain [25], was designed to overcome the limitations of a standard LMA as an intubating device. The principal features are an anatomically curved, rigid airway tube with an integral guiding handle. A 15 mm connector allows ventilation through this tube which will allow tracheal tube size of up to 8 mm. The anatomical curve permits insertion without head and neck manipulation or insertion of fingers in the mouth. A V-shaped tracheal tube guiding ramp helps to centralize the tracheal tube and guides it anteriorly to reduce risk of arytenoid trauma and oesophageal placement. An epiglottic elevating bar has replaced the LMA mask bars designed to protect and elevate the epiglottis during tracheal tube passage.

To avoid the problems of railroading with ordinary tubes, a proprietary tracheal tube is supplied with the device. This is made of silicone, is straight and reinforced and comes with a detachable 15 mm connector and a tip, with an offset distal opening, designed to avoid impingement of the tube on the vocal cords or arytenoids. A tracheal tube 'pusher' is also supplied with the kit for easier removal of the ILMA over the tracheal tube once intubation is complete.

The reported success rate of blind intubation through an ILMA in patients with normal airways varies between 93% and 99% [26–28]. In the UK multicentre study [27], 96% of the 500 patients were intubated within three attempts by experienced anaesthetists who were new to the ILMA. Insertion at first attempt was 79.8%, second attempt 12.4% and third attempt 4%. Of the 19 failures, 5 resulted from oesophageal intubation, in one case a narrow laryngeal opening was revealed and in one patient intubation was not attempted due to previous pharyngeal pouch surgery. Oesophageal perforation in a patient during blind placement has been reported [29]. Fibreoptic guidance is equally successful in intubating through the ILMA [30]. Although it takes slightly longer, a visual method with a fibrescope is preferred to avoid trauma to the upper airway, especially in patients with difficult airway (Figure 4.11).

Blind intubation through the ILMA has been reported in patients in whom intubation had previously failed and in whom difficult intubation was predicted [31,32]. Awake intubation has also been described through an ILMA [33]. Failure of ILMA in a patient with a large goitre has been reported [34]. This patient was subsequently intubated with a LMA-assisted fibreoptic intubation.

An ILMA-assisted fibreoptic guided intubation would be the best combination since the ILMA has all advantages of a LMA (see Table 5.2) and additionally its design avoids all the limitations of the standard LMA as an intubating device. Where possible, this device should be used in preference to LMA. At the present moment the device is expensive and many anaesthetists may not be experienced in its use although the learning curve is steep. One disadvantage of the ILMA is that it cannot safely be

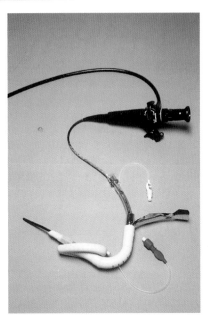

Figure 4.11   Intubating laryngeal mask airway (ILMA) with dedicated tube. Fibreoptic-guided tracheal intubation through ILMA is preferred to blind intubation

inserted when the mouth opening is less than 20 mm (LMA 11 mm). A lower success rate for both insertion and blind intubation has been shown when cricoid pressure is applied. The ILMA has not replaced direct laryngoscopy for routine intubation. There is concern that the process of intubation is blind, it is relatively costly and anaesthetists should have practice in using it on patients with normal airway before using it for patients with difficult airways.

Cuffed oropharyngeal airway

A modification of the Guedel airway, the cuffed oropharyngeal airway (COPA), provides hands-free anaesthesia and ventilation because the proximal portion of the airway can be connected to a breathing circuit and its distal pharyngeal portion has a cuff, which will provide an airtight seal. After induction, anaesthesia is maintained with the COPA in a spontaneously breathing patient or by gentle manual ventilation [35].

Orotracheal fibreoptic intubation through COPA

Direct technique

Unlike in the LMA, the lumen of the COPA is not wide enough to accept tracheal tubes of 6 mm. A technique of passing a fibrescope into the oral cavity so that its tip is guided along the side of the COPA and into the glottis has been described [36]. The COPA may have to be manipulated in the oropharynx and its cuff deflated. Once the tip of the fibrescope is in the trachea, the COPA is removed and the tracheal tube railroaded over the fibrescope. This is not a satisfactory technique and cannot be recommended. A similar technique for nasotracheal intubation is also possible.

Aintree Intubation Catheter technique (Figure 4.12)

Two-stage techniques are more satisfactory with COPA. An intubating fibrescope with a 4 mm insertion cord will easily pass through the lumen of the COPA. A technique using the Aintree

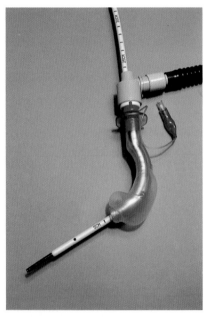

Figure 4.12 Aintree Intubation Catheter (AIC) assisted fibreoptic intubation through cuffed oropharyngeal airway (COPA). An intubating fibrescope loaded with an AIC will pass through a COPA. The COPA and fibrescope are removed and a suitable tracheal tube is railroaded over the AIC

Intubation Catheter similar to that used with a LMA has been described [37]. This technique has also been reported in a patient with a difficult airway [38].

● References

1. Ovassapian A. A new fibreoptic intubating airway. *Anesth Anal* 1987; **66 Suppl:** S132, p38.
2. Smith JE, Mackenzie AA, Scott Knight VCE. Comparison of two methods of fibrescope guided tracheal intubation. *Br J Anaesth* 1991; **66:** 546–50.
3. Berman RA. A method for blind intubation of the trachea or esophagus. *Anesth Analg* 1977; **56:** 866–7.
4. Patil V, Stehling LC, Zauder HL, Koch JP. Mechanical aids for fiberoptic endoscopy. *Anesthesiology* 1982; **57:** 69–70.
5. Higgins MS and Marco A. An aid in oral fibreoptic intubation. *Anesthesiology* 1992; **77:** 1236–7.
6. Coe PA, King TA, Towey RM. Teaching guided fibreoptic nasotracheal intubation. *Anaesthesia* 1988; **43:** 410–13.
7. Ralston SJ, Charters P. Cuffed nasopharyngeal tube as 'dedicated airway' in difficult intubation. *Anaesthesia* 1994; **49:** 133–6.
8. Nakan A. Blind tracheal intubation through laryngeal mask. *J Clin Anesth* 1992; **16:** 657–8.
9. Heath ML, Allegain J. The Brain Laryngeal Mask as an aid to intubation. *Anaesthesia* 1991; **46:** 545–8.
10. Lim SL, Tay DHB, Thomas E. A comparison of three types of tracheal tube for use in laryngeal mask assisted blind oropharyngeal intubation. *Anaesthesia* 1994; **49:** 255–7.
11. Benumof JL. The laryngeal mask airway and the ASA difficult airway algorithm. *Anesthesiology* 1996; **84:** 686–99.
12. Preis CA, Hartmann T, Zimpfer M. Laryngeal mask airway facilitates awake fibreoptic intubation in a patient with severe oropharyngeal bleeding. *Anesth Analg* 1998; **87:** 728–9.
13. Osborne WA, Jackson AP, Smith JE. The laryngeal mask airway as an aid to training in fibreoptic nasotracheal endoscopy. *Anaesthesia* 1998; **53:** 1080–83.
14. Charters P, O'Sullivan E. The 'dedicated airway' : a review of the concept and an update of current practice. *Anaesthesia* 1999; **54:** 778–86.
15. Asai T, Latto IP, Vaughan RS. The distance between the grille of the laryngeal mask and the vocal cords. *Anaesthesia* 1993; **48:** 667.
16. Asai TA. Tracheal intubation through the LMA. *Anesthesiology* 1996; **84:** 439.
17. Reynold PI, O'Kelly SW. Fiberoptic intubation and the laryngeal mask airway. *Anesthesiology* 1993; **79:** 1144.
18. Koga K, Asai T, Latto IP, Vaughan RS. Effect of the size of a tracheal tube and the efficacy of the use of the laryngeal mask for fibrescope-aided tracheal intubation. *Anaesthesia* 1997; **52:** 131–5.
19. Kadota Y, Oda T, Yoshimura N. Application of a laryngeal mask to a fibreoptic bronchoscope-aided tracheal intubation. *J Clin Anesth* 1992; **4:** 503–4.

20. Darling JR, Keohane M, Murray JMA. A split laryngeal mask as an aid to training in fiberoptic tracheal intubation. *Anaesthesia* 1993; **48:** 1079–82.
21. Atherton DPL, O'Sullivan E, Lowe D, Charters P. A ventilation-exchange bougie for fibreoptic intubations with the laryngeal mask airway. *Anaesthesia* 1996; **51:** 1123–6.
22. Allison A, McCrory J. Tracheal placement of a gum-elastic bougie using the LMA. *Anaesthesia* 1990; **45:** 419–20.
23. Sartore DM, Kojima RK.Laryngeal mask airway assisted wire-guided fibreoptic tracheal intubation. *Anesthesiology* 1994; **81:** 1550–51.
24. Alexander R, Moore C. The laryngeal mask airway and training in naso-tracheal intubation. *Anaesthesia* 1993; **48:** 350–51.
25. Brain AIJ et al. The ILMA II: a preliminary clinical report of a new means of intubating the trachea. *Br J Anaesth* 1997; **79:**704–9.
26. Kapila A, Addy EV, Verghese C, Brain Al. The ILMA: an initial assessment of performance. *Br J Anaesth* 1997; **79:** 710–13.
27. Baskett PJ, Parr MJ, Nolan JP. The intubating laryngeal mask. Results of a multicentre trial with experience of 500 cases. *Anaesthesia* 1998; **53:** 1174–9.
28. Agro F, Brimacombe J, Carassiti M, Marchionni L, Cataldo R. The intubating laryngeal mask. Clinical appraisal of ventilation and blind tracheal intubation in 110 patients. *Anaesthesia* 1998; **53:** 1084–90.
29. Branthwaite MA. An unexpected complication of the intubating laryngeal mask. *Anaesthesia* 1999; **54:** 166–71.
30. Joo HS, Rose DK. The intubating laryngeal mask with and without fibreoptic guidance. *Anesth Analg* 1999; **88:** 662–6.
31. Parr MJA, Gregory M, Baskett PJF. The intubating laryngeal mask. Use in difficult or failed intubation. *Anaesthesia* 1998; **53:** 343–8.
32. Joo H, Rose K. Fast trach – a new intubating laryngeal mask airway; successful use in patients with difficult airways. *Can J Anaesth* 1998; **45;** 1222–3.
33. Asai T, Matsumato H, Shingu K. Awake tracheal intubation through the intubating laryngeal mask. *Can J Anaesth* 1999; **46:** 182–4.
34. Wakeling HG, Ody A, Ball A. Large goiter causing difficult intubation and failure to intubate using the intubating laryngeal airway: lessons for next time. *Br J Anaesth* 1998; **81:** 979–81.
35. Asai T, Koga K, Jones RM, Stacey M et al. The cuffed oropharyngeal airway. Its clinical use in 100 patients. *Anaesthesia* 1998; **53:** 81–2.
36. Greenberg RS, Kay NH. Cuffed oropharyngeal airway (COPA) as an adjunct to fibreoptic tracheal intubation. *Br J Anaesth* 1999; **82:** 395–8.
37. Hawkins M, O'Sullivan E, Charters P. Fibreoptic intubation using the cuffed oropharyngeal airway and Aintree catheter. *Anaesthesia* 1998; **53:** 891–4.
38. Hawkins M, Roberts EA. Use of a cuffed oropharyngeal airway and Aintree catheter in a difficult airway. *Anaesthesia* 1999; **54:** 909–10.

5

Fibreoptic intubation in difficult airway management

• Introduction

Difficulty in maintaining a patent airway and placing a tracheal tube in an anaesthetized patient has always been a cause of concern to anaesthetists. These difficulties can sometimes lead to morbidity and mortality. Exact figures are unknown, but data from the American Closed Claims Study showed that difficult intubation claims accounted for 17% of the total adverse respiratory claims; 75% of these were preventable or due to substandard care and 85% resulted in death or brain death [1]. In the UK, the first *Report of a Confidential Enquiry into Perioperative Deaths* stated that one in three anaesthetic-related deaths was due to failure to intubate the trachea [2]. Two approaches may improve this situation. First, optimizing preoperative predictors of anticipating difficulties in intubation and/or mask ventilation. Second, introducing safe and effective techniques to manage patients when difficulty (anticipated or unanticipated) is encountered.

For the first approach to succeed, predictors of difficult intubation should have a high sensitivity (percentage of correctly predicted difficult intubations as a proportion of all intubations that were truly difficult) and specificity (percentage of correctly predicted easy intubations as a proportion of all intubations that were truly easy). None of the tests, some described in this chapter, performed singly or in combination, can achieve this ideal. The second approach, of optimizing the safe and effective management of a patient with a difficult airway, whether anticipated or not, therefore assumes an even greater importance.

Many new devices and techniques have been introduced to achieve intubation in patients presenting with a difficult airway [3]. When faced with a difficult situation, anaesthetists should use techniques and devices with which they are most familiar. Difficult airway management is one such situation. Of the many airway devices introduced in the last few years, the laryngeal mask airway (LMA) has made the biggest impact as a ventilatory device. The flexible fibrescope has revolutionized the management of patients with known anatomical difficulties in tracheal intubation [4]. The application of flexible fibreoptic intubation for difficult airway management, including the possible role of LMA-assisted fibreoptic intubation, are discussed in this chapter. It is hoped that anaesthetists will then appreciate that the flexible fibrescope is the one intubating device that they should become most familiar with for management of patients with a difficult airway.

● Definition of terms

Difficult airway

This is the clinical situation in which a conventionally trained anaesthesiologist experiences difficulty with mask ventilation, difficulty with tracheal intubation or both. This definition was introduced by the American Society of Anesthesiologists (ASA) Task Force on management of the difficult airway [5].

Failed intubation

This is defined as the inability to place an endotracheal tube. It has a definite end-point and therefore its reporting in the literature is uniform. The incidence in the general population is 0.05% or about 1:2230 and approximately 0.13–0.35% or 1:750–1:280 in the obstetric population [6].

Difficult endotracheal intubation

The ASA Task Force defined this as 'the proper insertion of an endotracheal tube with conventional laryngoscopy that requires more than three attempts, more than 10 minutes or both'. This definition is inappropriate because an experienced anaesthetist may be able to identify a difficult intubation at the first attempt and within 30 seconds. The concept of optimal or best attempt at laryngoscopy was introduced to overcome some of the problems with this definition [7]. Anaesthetists should achieve their best attempt at laryngoscopy as early as possible and if this fails than a second back-up plan (plan B) should be activated without further risk to the patient. A best or optimal attempt at laryngoscopy would include:

1. Performance by a reasonably experienced anaesthetist.
2. Use of optimal sniffing position.
3. Use of optimal external laryngeal manipulation (OELM).
4. One change in the length of the blade.
5. One change in the type of the blade.

With the sequence of these events, the optimal or best attempt at laryngoscopy can be achieved at the first attempt and should not take more than four attempts. Another definition of difficult intubation has been proposed as follows [8]: When an experienced laryngoscopist, using direct laryngoscopy, requires

- more than two attempts with the same blade, or
- a change in the blade or an adjunct to a direct laryngoscope (e.g. bougie), or
- use of an alternative device or technique following failed intubation with direct laryngoscopy.

This definition is independent of time and number of attempts and probably comes close to covering the clinical realities of difficulties for everyone [9].

Difficult laryngoscopy

This is defined as a laryngoscopy in which it is not possible to see any of the vocal cords when using a conventional laryngoscope and would equate to a Cormack and Lehane grade 3 or 4 [10] (Figure 5.1).

Difficult mask ventilation

This occurs when it is not possible for the unassisted anaesthesiologist to prevent reversal of signs of inadequate ventilation and to maintain oxygen saturation greater than 90% using 100% oxygen and positive pressure ventilation in a patient with preoperative saturation greater than 90%.

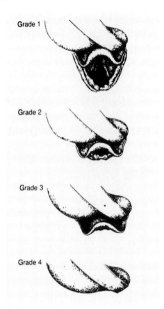

Figure 5.1   Cormack and Lehane classification of direct laryngoscopy grades. A 'difficult' laryngoscopy is one in which it is not possible to see any of the vocal cords and would equate to grade 3 and 4 (From K.N. Williams, F. Carli and R.S. Cormack (1991) Unexpected difficult laryngoscopy: a prospective survey in routine general surgery. *British Journal of Anaesthesia*; **66:** 38–44 © The Board of Management and Trustees of the *British Journal of Anaesthesia*. Reproduced by permission of Oxford University Press/*British Journal of Anaesthesia*.)

Incidence of difficult airway

It has not been possible to work out the exact incidence of difficult airway because of the problems in defining the various end-points. Table 5.1 gives a very rough estimate to understand the frequency with which each scenario occurs in the general population.

● Prediction and causes of difficult laryngoscopy

It is important to take a full history, and perform a general examination and specific airway assessment in most cases. In many instances the airway is grossly abnormal and difficulty is quickly predicted, but a careful assessment must be performed to

Table 5.1   Incidence of difficult airway in the general population (not obstetrics)

Difficult laryngoscopy (grades 3–4)	10%	1:10
Difficult intubation	1%	1:100
Failed intubation	0.05%	1:2000
Can't ventilate	0.01–0.03%	1–3:10 000

make an airway management plan. Occasionally, there may not be enough time to conduct a full examination, but the nature of the patient's condition will be a cause for suspicion. The previous anaesthetic notes should be sought and checked.

History

The patient can give important information about previous airway difficulty. The previous anaesthetist may have given details to the patient who may have a note or a bracelet. This may give information about techniques previously used.

General examination

General examination of the patient may help in identifying systemic disease or pathology that may be associated with airway difficulty such as obesity, scleroderma, rheumatoid arthritis, acromegaly and so on. Altered mental status, hypertension and tachycardia (due to hypoxaemia and hypercarbia) may suggest airway obstruction. The breathing pattern may help in identifying the site and extent of obstruction; prolonged inspiration and stridor may be present when there is critical upper airway obstruction, prolonged expiration when there is lower airway obstruction. Subcutaneous emphysema may be present in airway distortion and there may be voice changes due to pathology at the level of the glottis.

Specific airway assessment

The procedure of direct laryngoscopy and intubation with a Macintosh blade involves bringing the axis of the oral cavity, pharynx and larynx in the same line. This is achieved when

- The neck is flexed (bringing the pharyngeal and laryngeal axis in line).
- The head is extended (bringing the oral axis in line with the other two axes).
- The mouth is adequately opened (to insert the laryngoscope blade).
- The tongue is displaced (to manoeuvre the blade from the right side of the mouth).
- The tongue and mandible are displaced anteriorly (to slip the blade in the vallecula and under the epiglottis).
- The tracheal tube is guided through the laryngeal inlet under vision.

These requirements are achieved when the following anatomical structures and their functions are within 'normal' limits:

- Normal flexion of the neck.
- Normal extension of the atlas on the occiput.
- Normal temporomandibular joint (mouth opening).
- Normal forward movement of the mandible and tongue.
- Normal anatomy of upper airway.

Many tests designed to anticipate airway difficulties have been described and reviewed in the literature [11]. A simple scheme based on the assessment of the anatomical structures and their function is presented below. The 'Causes' information indicates the causes of deviation from normal anatomy or function.

Function:	Flexion of the neck.
Test:	Ask the patient to flex the neck to 90° (the first component of the 'sniffing the morning air' position).
Function:	Normal extension of the occiput on the atlas.
Test:	Examine the patient from the side and ask them to adopt the position of 'sniffing the morning air' – flexion of cervical spine and extension of the head on the neck.
Causes:	Bony deformities as in rheumatoid arthritis, ankylosis, cervical spine trauma. Soft-tissue pathology as in short and bull neck, obesity, large goitre or other mass in the neck.
Function:	Normal temporomandibular joint.
Test:	Mouth opening: the patient should be able to insert three fingers (4 cm) between the teeth.
Causes:	Temporomandibular joint disease, e.g. systemic causes like rheumatoid arthritis; localized pathology causing trismus, e.g. ankylosis, infection, tumour, irradiation.
Function:	Normal forward movement of the mandible and tongue.
Test:	Ask the patient to bring the lower teeth in front of the upper teeth.

Causes: Maxillary overbite (buck teeth) or micrognathia (e.g. congenital syndromes such as Pierre Robin or Treacher Collins, juvenile rheumatoid arthritis) or a fixed mandible (tumour, infection, trauma or irradiation).

Function: Normal anatomy of oral cavity and pharynx.

Test: Mallampati (or Samsoon and Young modification) tests. These tests determine the relative tongue/pharyngeal size and are conducted by inspection of the back of the mouth as follows. With the head in the neutral position, the patient opens the mouth wide and protrudes the tongue as far as possible. Sitting opposite the patient, the anaesthetist then examines the back of the mouth.

   Mallampati [12] described three classes and Samsoon and Young [13] added a fourth one. This test forms the basis of assessing the size of the tongue in relation to the size of the oral cavity (Figure 5.2):

   Class I   = soft palate, fauces, uvula, anterior and posterior pillars
   Class II = soft palate, fauces, uvula
   Class III = soft palate, base of uvula
   Class IV = soft palate not visible at all

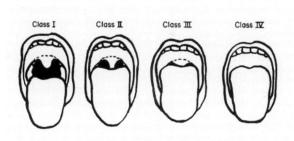

Figure 5.2 Samsoon and Young classification of relative tongue/pharyngeal size to predict difficult laryngoscopy. See text for details (From Samsoon and Young [13] with permission from Blackwell Science)

Most anaesthetists would consider that patients with a class III or IV airway would have a difficult laryngoscopy.

Causes: Reduced mandibular space causing relative macroglossia due to micrognathia (see above) or absolute macroglossia (e.g. Down's syndrome and acromegaly). Abnormal anatomy causing airway compromise (tumour, infection, irradiation, trauma, surgery or congenital causes).

Thyromental distance – Patil distance [14]

The distance between the tip of the mandible and the anterior aspect of the thyroid cartilage is normally 6.5 cm. A distance of less than 6 cm may be associated with difficult intubation.

Sternomental distance – Savva distance [15]

The distance between the tip of the mandible and the sternal notch. In a normal adult this distance is 12.5 cm. A distance of less than 12 cm may be associated with difficult intubation.

Other tests

The above tests may not identify airway difficulties due to glottic or subglottic pathology where the history is most important. Other tests such as X-rays, CT and MRI scans of the upper airway and chest, blood gas analysis and pulmonary function tests may aid in evaluation of the airway. In cases of airway obstruction, results of an upper airway endoscopy examination performed by an ENT surgeon may help in planning the management.

In many clinical situations, a full airway assessment may not be possible because the condition of the patient requires urgent resuscitation. The airway difficulty is usually obvious or there is a high degree of suspicion. Some examples include patients with maxillofacial trauma, stridor due to upper airway obstruction (trauma, tumour, infection and burns), and bleeding in the oral cavity (bleeding tonsil or trauma). In some patients difficulty at laryngoscopy and intubation is seen unexpectedly despite all the tests being normal.

● Role of fibreoptic intubation in difficult airway management

Efforts have been made in the last 10 years, particularly in the USA, to provide guidelines on difficult airway management with the help of algorithms [5]. The ASA algorithm stresses the importance of recognition of difficult airway and proper preparation for its management and guides the clinician on the management options when faced with a difficult airway under different circumstances. The full description of the algorithm and the management options are beyond the scope of this chapter. The latest modifications of the ASA algorithm are reviewed by Benumof [7].

Table 5.2 shows the clinical scenarios in which a patient with a difficult airway may present and the management options for ventilation and/or intubation in this scenario. The last column indicates the fibreoptic technique that may be appropriate to that scenario.

Table 5.2 Role of fibreoptic intubation in difficult airway management

Clinical scenario	Management options (ventilation/ intubation)	Flexible fibreoptic intubation (FFI) technique
1. Anticipated difficult airway	Awake intubation choices*	Awake FFI
2. Anticipated difficult airway but awake intubation not feasible	Intubation choices under GA†	FFI with conduit airway, LMA or ILMA
3. Unanticipated difficult laryngoscopy during routine induction – can't intubate, can ventilate	Intubation choices under GA†	FFI with conduit airway, LMA or ILMA
4. Unanticipated difficult airway during rapid sequence induction (failed intubation)	Mask ventilation, LMA Awaken patient	? FFI with LMA Awake FFI
5. Unanticipated difficult airway – can't ventilate can't intubate	LMA, Combitube, transtracheal jet ventilation (TTJV)	? FFI with LMA

*Awake intubation choices: awake flexible fibreoptic intubation, awake direct laryngoscopy, awake blind intubation, awake retrograde intubation or awake surgical airway.

†**Intubation choices under general anaesthesia**: different laryngoscope blades, gum elastic bougie, flexible fibreoptic intubation, lightwand, retrograde intubation or surgical airway.

Airway management plan

The following are essential prerequisites to a successful outcome in the management of a difficult intubation scenario with any device or technique:

- Airway assessment and proper preparation of the patient.
- Skilled anaesthetist.
- Proper equipment available.
- Skilled assistance.
- Back-up plan (plan B) worked out *before* primary technique (plan A) is started.

The reason for the possible application of flexible fibreoptic instruments in many of the difficult airway scenarios is because of certain characteristics that make them 'ideal' intubating devices. These are summarized in Table 5.3.

Table 5.3   Characteristics of flexible fibreoptic instruments making them ideal intubating devices

Flexibility conforms easily to normal and difficult airway anatomy

Continuous visualization of airway during endoscopy

Less traumatic than rigid laryngoscope

Latest equipment is lightweight and portable

Can be used with other intubating techniques (e.g. direct laryngoscopy)

Can be used with ventilatory devices (e.g. LMA)

Can be used for oral or nasal intubation

Can be used on patients of all age groups

Definitive check of tube position in trachea

Ability to use camera and monitor for teaching

Clinical scenario 1: anticipated difficult airway

Benumof has suggested that if it is recognized that intubation or mask ventilation is going to be difficult because of the presence of a pathological factor or a combination of anatomical factors (large tongue size, small mandibular space, or restricted atlanto-occipital extension), then the airway patency should be secured and guaranteed (usually by intubation) while the patient remains awake [6]. In simple terms, a difficult direct laryngoscopy can be expected if it is doubtful that the oral cavity, pharynx and trachea can be brought in a straight line (see 'Prediction and causes of difficult laryngoscopy', earlier). In this situation the airway should be secured while the patient is awake for the following reasons (Figure 5.3 a–c):

■ The natural airway is preserved (intact pharyngeal muscle tone).
■ Spontaneous breathing is maintained (oxygenation and ventilation).
■ An awake patient is easier to intubate (the larynx moves forward with general anaesthesia).
■ The patient can protect his/her airway from aspiration of gastric contents.
■ Patients' neurological status can be monitored (e.g. unstable cervical spine).

Compared with other choices for awake intubation (see Table 5.2), such as awake direct laryngoscopy, awake retrograde and awake blind intubation, awake flexible fibreoptic intubation in experienced hands has the following advantages:

■ Excellent patient acceptability.
■ Ability to apply topical anaesthetic and insufflate oxygen during intubation.
■ Very high success rate.
■ Less cardiovascular changes during awake intubation than with rigid laryngoscope intubation.

Awake flexible fibreoptic intubation has been used in a number of conditions associated with a difficult airway (see 'Clinical application', below), but may not be the technique of choice for all patients with an anticipated difficult airway. Some limitations of its use are:

■ Massive bleeding in the upper airway (Figure 5.4).
■ Laryngeal/tracheal disruption.
■ Combined maxillary and mandibular fractures.
■ Upper airway obstruction at glottic level (see Chapter 9).
■ Uncooperative patient (see under 'Clinical scenario 2', below)

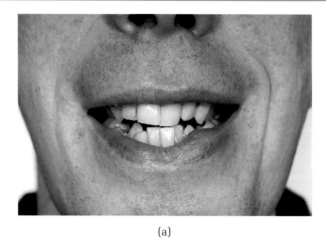

(a)

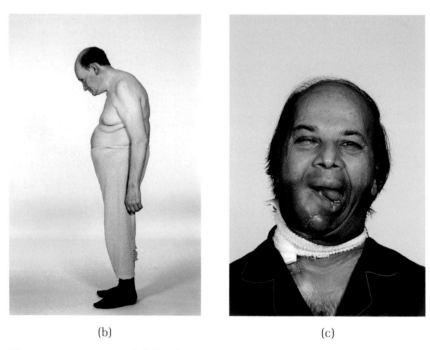

(b)   (c)

Figure 5.3   Anticipated difficult airway: (a) limited mouth opening due to temporomandibular joint disease; (b) severe cervical spine flexion deformity due to ankylosing spondylitis; (c) limited mouth opening due to previous oral cancer surgery and radiotherapy. In all cases, direct laryngoscopy would be impossible due to failure to get the oral pharyngeal and tracheal axis in a straight line. Awake nasotracheal fibreoptic intubation was easily accomplished in all cases

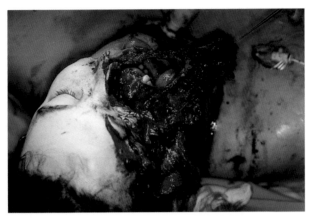

Figure 5.4 Massive bleeding in the oral cavity is a contraindication for fibreoptic intubation. This patient with bilateral maxillary fractures was easy to intubate with a Macintosh laryngoscope. A tracheostomy was then performed for surgical access

Clinical scenario 2: anticipated difficult airway but awake intubation not feasible (Figure 5.5)

This scenario includes some young children and adults who may not cooperate during awake intubation; for example, patients with learning difficulties, altered conscious level and language difficulties (Figure 5.5a,b). Anaesthesia may be conducted with a ventilatory device such as a LMA. If intubation is required, then fibreoptic intubation under general anaesthesia is a safe and practical option. Depending on individual assessment, induction of anaesthesia may be intravenous or gaseous, but muscle relaxation should not be instituted before manual ventilation with bag and mask is confirmed and the ability to ventilate manually is guaranteed. Fibreoptic intubation may be performed through any of the conduit airways. A LMA-assisted or an ILMA-assisted fibreoptic intubation is another option with its added advantages (see Chapters 4 and 6).

Clinical scenario 3: unanticipated difficult laryngoscopy during routine induction – can't intubate, can ventilate

In this clinical scenario, difficulty in intubation is recognized only after induction of anaesthesia. The patient is usually paralysed with a non-depolarizing muscle relaxant. Intubation is difficult, but it is usually possible to ventilate the patient's lungs

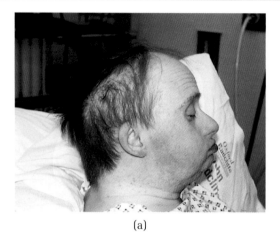

(a)

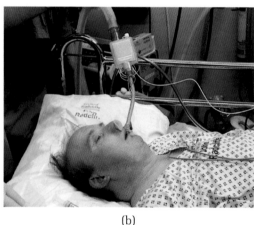

(b)

Figure 5.5 Anticipated difficult airway – awake fibreoptic intubation not feasible: (a) Down's syndrome with micrognathia, macroglossia and previous documented grade 4 laryngoscopy but easy mask ventilation; (b) successfully intubated with a LMA-assisted fibreoptic intubation using an Aintree Intubation Catheter (see Chapter 4 for details of technique)

with a bag and mask. An option is to perform fibreoptic intubation under general anaesthesia. Any of the conduit airways or a LMA or an ILMA can be used to assist fibreoptic intubation (see Chapter 4). One danger of persistent attempts at intubation using a variety of blades and the gum elastic bougie is the trauma, oedema and bleeding that is caused to the upper airway. Eventually an airway that could be managed by mask ventilation becomes an unmanageable airway. This sequence of events has been repeatedly highlighted in closed claims where patients have become hypoxic with repeated intubation attempts.

An anaesthetist experienced in performing fibreoptic intubation should use it as an early option in the airway management plan. This will ensure high success rate and avoid subsequent trauma to the upper airway. This is crucial because if fibreoptic intubation is considered late, there is every chance that it may fail due to the presence of blood and secretions. Ovassapian has confirmed the role of fibreoptic intubation in this scenario (see 'Clinical application', below). It is likely that application of fibreoptic intubation in this scenario will increase with the increase and availability of portable equipment.

Clinical scenario 4: unanticipated difficult intubation during rapid sequence induction (failed intubation)

The priorities in this clinical scenario are to keep the patient oxygenated and at the same time prevent aspiration of gastric contents by maintaining cricoid pressure. The problems of maintaining adequate ventilation with a facemask and LMA in the presence of continuous cricoid pressure are well known [16,17]. Although cricoid pressure must be maintained to prevent aspiration, oxygenation should always be the first priority. In the presence of difficulty with mask ventilation, insertion of a LMA is recommended. A controlled release of cricoid pressure is allowed to facilitate insertion of and ventilation through a LMA, if this is difficult [18,19]. The options are to continue general anaesthesia using a LMA or awaken the patient. If the patient is woken up, then an awake flexible fibreoptic intubation is the technique of choice. It is possible that an anaesthetist skilled in fibreoptic intubation would be able to intubate the trachea in a few seconds through the LMA. There are no reports of the use of a LMA in this situation, but the ILMA has been successfully used in two patients requiring rapid sequence induction for cervical spine injury [20].

Initial trials using conduit airways (see Chapter 4) are promising and have shown that the technique is practically feasible [21, 22]. One assistant maintains the cricoid pressure and another applies jaw thrust while the anaesthetist performs the endoscopy and intubation. The problems with the technique are that two assistants are required and the equipment should be at hand (portable fibrescopes are very useful) (see Figure 5.6). The time taken for fibreoptic intubation is longer than conven-

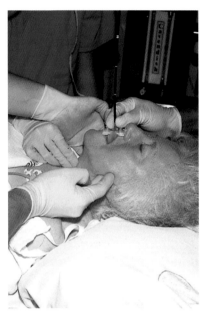

Figure 5.6 Rapid sequence fibreoptic intubation. One assistant applies cricoid pressure and another jaw thrust, while the anaesthetist performs orotracheal fibreoptic intubation through a conduit airway

tional laryngoscopy, but clinically patients come to no harm [22]. One useful aspect of this technique is that cricoid pressure applied incorrectly and causing airway obstruction can easily be identified endoscopically [23]. If a LMA has been used for rescue ventilation, it is a perfect conduit and ventilatory device for fibreoptic intubation (see Chapter 4).

It is clear that more work is needed before fibreoptic intubation can be recommended in this scenario. Because of the increasing use of fibrescopes by anaesthetists and the availability of portable equipment, it is likely that there would be increasing use of this technique in the future.

Clinical scenario 5: unanticipated difficult airway – can't ventilate, can't intubate

This clinical scenario is every anaesthetist's nightmare. The priority is maintaining ventilation of the patient. The ASA algorithm has recommended airway devices such as LMA and Combitube for maintaining ventilation [7]. If ventilation with these devices is successful, a decision can be made to wake up the patient if a short-acting muscle relaxant has been used. An awake fibreoptic intubation can then be performed. Alternatively a decision may be made to continue anaesthesia using a LMA. A third option is to perform a LMA-assisted fibreoptic intubation [24]. A transtracheal jet ventilation cannula should be introduced without delay if ventilation through a LMA is inadequate [7].

● Clinical application of fibreoptic techniques in difficult airway management

The first flexible fibreoptic-guided tracheal intubation was described by Dr Peter Murphy in 1967 [25]. Five years after the publication of his report, almost in the space of a few weeks, two separate reports of the use of a fibreoptic bronchoscope for awake intubation appeared from both sides of the Atlantic [26,27]. Stiles and colleagues reported a series of 100 fibreoptic intubations with 4 failures. They commented that 20 of their patients would have had difficult laryngoscopy and another 34 would have required tracheostomy under local anaesthesia [28]. In 1974, Davis described an awake fibreoptic intubation for a patient with ankylosing spondylitis [29]. In the same year, Prithvi Raj and colleagues described 50 patients, in 30 of whom nasal/oral fibreoptic intubation was achieved under topical anaesthesia, cricothyroid puncture and sedation [30]. Masseter and Petersson compared 41 consecutive patients suffering from severe rheumatoid arthritis having conventional direct laryngoscopy or flexible fibreoptic intubation and found that the latter technique significantly reduced the number of complicated intubations [31]. Since these early reports, flexible fibreoptic intubation has been used in numerous conditions where difficulty in intubation is anticipated. Its application has been extended to the management of patients in differing clinical situations such as in trauma [32], cervical spine disease [33], in children [34] and in patients at risk of aspiration [35] and obstetrics [36].

Ovassapian has confirmed the safety and efficacy of fibreoptic intubation in difficult airway management. Within a total of 2031 fibreoptic intubations between 1978 and 1989 in his institution, there were 302 patients with anatomical and or pathological conditions rendering the use of rigid laryngoscopy difficult or impossible. On these 302 patients, 338 intubations

Table 5.4 Categories of difficult intubation (From Ovassapian [37] with permission from Lippincott, Williams and Wilkins)

Category	Common causes*	Compromised airway†	Total
Anticipated difficult airway			
Physical findings	47	147	194
History of difficult or failed intubation	69	42	111
Unanticipated difficult intubation			
Failed rigid intubation followed by fibreoptic intubation attempts	28	5	33
Total	144	194	338

*Common causes. Combination of features such as short thick neck, limited neck extension, protruding incisors, large tongue, narrow mouth-opening, receding mandible, marked obesity, high arched palate

†Compromised airway. Patients with anatomical abnormalities of the head, neck or upper airway, resulting from surgery, radiation, burn scars, tumours, trauma, infection, arthritis, ankylosing spondylitis of the cervical spine and diseases such as scleroderma and acromegaly.

were performed [37] (Table 5.4). In 305 of the 338 occasions, difficult tracheal intubation was expected due to physical findings or because of a history of previous difficult/failed intubation. In the remaining 33 cases tracheal intubation using the rigid technique had failed unexpectedly during general anaesthesia and fibreoptic intubation was required.

Fibreoptic intubation was attempted on 287 occasions with the patient awake but sedated, with local anaesthetic applied to the airway. In 51 patients the airway was intubated after induction of general anaesthesia. Fibreoptic intubation was successful in 334 out of 338 attempts (98.8%).

In summary, these data confirm the role of fibreoptic intubation in the clinical scenarios of anticipated difficult airway and in unanticipated difficult intubation after induction of anaesthesia when conventional laryngoscopy has failed.

● **References**

1. Cheyney FW, Posner KL, Caplan RA. Adverse respiratory events infrequently leading to malpractice suits. A closed claims analysis. *Anesthesiology* 1991; **75**: 932–9.
2. Buck N, Devlin HB, Lunn JN. *The Report of a Confidential Enquiry into Perioperative Deaths* NCEPOD, London, 1987.
3. Latto IP. Management of difficult intubation. In: Latto IP and Vaughn RS eds. *Difficulties in Tracheal Intubation*, 2nd edn, pp. 107–60. WB Saunders, London, 1997.
4. Gaba DM. Anaesthesiology as a model for patient safety in health care. *Br Med J* 2000; **320**: 785–8.
5. Caplan RA et al. Practice Guidelines for Management of the Difficult Airway. A report by the American Society of Anesthesiologists Task Force on management of the difficult airway. *Anesthesiology* 1993; **78**: 597–602.
6. Benumof JL. Management of the difficult airway: with special emphasis on awake tracheal intubation. *Anesthesiology* 1991; **75**: 1087–110.
7. Benumof JL. ASA Difficult airway algorithm: new thoughts and considerations. In: Hagberg CA ed. *Handbook of Difficult Airway Management*, pp. 31–48. Churchill Livingstone, Philadelphia, 2000.
8. Crosby ET, Cooper RM, Diyghlas MJ et al. The unanticipated difficult airway with recommendations for management. *Can J Anaesth* 1998; **45**: 757–76.
9. Benumof JL. The unanticipated difficult airway. *Can J Anaesth*; 1999; **46**: 510.
10. Cormack RS and Lehane J. Difficult tracheal intubation in obstetrics. *Anaesthesia* 1984; **39**: 1105–11.
11. Wheeler M., Ovassapian A. Prediction and evaluation of the difficult airway. In: Hagberg CA ed. *Handbook of Difficult Airway Management*, pp. 15–30. Churchill Livingstone, Philadelphia, 2000.
12. Mallampati SR, Gatt SP, Gugino LD et al. A clinical sign to predict difficult tracheal intubation: a prospective study. *Can Anaesth Soc J* 1985; **32**: 429–34.
13. Samsoon GLT, Young JRB. Difficult tracheal intubation: a retrospective study. *Anaesthesia* 1987; **42**: 487–90.
14. Patil UV, Stehling LC, Zauder HL. Predicting the difficulty of tracheal intubation utilizing an intubation guide. *Anesthesiol Rev* 1983; **10**: 32.
15. Savva D. Prediction of difficult tracheal intubation. *Br J Anesth* 1994; **73**: 149.
16. Allman KG. The effect of cricoid pressure application on airway patency. *Journal of Clinical Anesthesia* 1995; **7**: 198–9.
17. Asai T, Barclay K, McBeth C, Vaughan RS. Cricoid pressure applied after placement of laryngeal mask prevents gastric insufflation but inhibits ventilation. *Br J Anaesth* 1996; **76**: 772–6.
18. Brimacombe JR, Berry AM. Cricoid pressure. *Can J Anaesth* 1997; **44**: 414–25.
19. Vanner RG, Asai T. Safe use of cricoid pressure. *Anesthesiology* 1999; **54**: 1–3.
20. Schuschnig C, Waltl B, Erlacher W, Reddy B et al. Intubating laryngeal mask and rapid sequence induction in patients with cervical spine injury. *Anaesthesia* 1999; **54**: 793–7.

21. Dravid RM, Pandit JJ, Iyer R, Popat M. Fibreoptic intubation for rapid sequence induction. *Europ J Anaesth* 2000; **17:** 65.
22. Ovassapian A, Krejcie TC, Joshi CW. Fibreoptic vs. rigid laryngoscopy for rapid sequence intubation of the trachea. *Anesth Analg* 1992; **74:** S229.
23. Palmer JH, Ball DR. The effect of cricoid pressure on the cricoid cartilage and vocal cords: an endoscopic study in anaesthetised patients. *Anesthesiology* 2000; **55:** 263–7.
24. Benumof JL. Use of the laryngeal mask airway to facilitate fibreoptic-aided tracheal intubation. *Anesth Analg* 1992; 74: 313–14.
25. Murphy P. A fiberoptic endoscope used for nasal intubation. *Anaesthesia* 1967; **22:** 489–91.
26. Taylor PA, Towey RM. The broncho-fiberscope as an aid to endotracheal intubation. *Br J Anaesth* 1972; **44:** 611–12.
27. Conyers AB, Wallace DH, Mulder DS. Use of the fiberoptic bronchoscope for nasotracheal intubation: a case report. *Can Anaesth Soc J* 1972; **19:** 654–6.
28. Stiles CM, Stiles QR, Denson JS. A flexible fiberoptic laryngoscope. *JAMA* 1972; **221:** 1246–7.
29. Davis NJ. A new fiberoptic laryngoscope for nasal intubation. *Anesth Analg* 1974; **52:** 807–8.
30. Prithvi Raj P, Forestner J, Watson TD et al. Techniques for fiberoptic laryngoscopy in anesthesia. *Anesth Analg* 1974; **53:** 708–14.
31. Masseter KH, Petersson KI. Endotracheal intubation with the fibreoptic bronchoscope. *Anaesthesia* 1980; **35:** 294–8.
32. Mulder DS, Wallace DH, Woolhouse FM. The use of the fiberoptic bronchoscope to facilitate endotracheal intubation following head and neck trauma. *J Trauma* 1975; **15:** 638–40.
33. Sidhu V, Whitehead EM, Ainsworth QP, Smith M, Calder I. A technique of awake intubation. Experience in patients with cervical spine disease. *Anesthesiology* 1993; **48:** 910–13.
34. Rucker RW, Silva WJ, Worchester CC. Fiberoptic bronchoscopic naso-tracheal intubation in children. *Chest* 1979; **76:** 56–8.
35. Ovassapian A, Krejcie TC, Yelich SJ, Dykes MH. Awake fibreoptic intubation in the patient at high risk of aspiration. *Br J Anaesth* 1989; **62:** 13–16.
36. Popat MT, Chippa JH, Russell R. Awake fibreoptic intubation following failed regional anaesthesia for Caesarean section in a parturient with Still's disease. *Eur J Anaesth* 2000; **17:** 211–14.
37. Ovassapian A. Fibreoptic tracheal intubation in adults. In: Ovassapian A ed. *Fibreoptic Endoscopy and the Difficult Airway*, 2nd edn, pp. 72–103. Lippincott-Raven, Philadelphia, 1996.

6

Fibreoptic intubation in the anaesthetized adult patient

- Indications and contraindications for fibreoptic intubation in anaesthetized patients
- Teaching fibreoptic intubation in anaesthetized patients
- Upper airway anatomy through the fibrescope
- Tracheal tube selection for fibreoptic intubation
- Techniques of teaching fibreoptic intubation in anaesthetized patients
- Teaching practical fibreoptic techniques under general anaesthesia
- Teaching oral fibreoptic intubation in anaesthetized patients
- Fibreoptic intubation under general anaesthesia in the difficult airway patient

● Indications and contraindications for fibreoptic intubation in anaesthetized patients

Indications

- Teaching and training in patients with a normal airway.
- Enhancing experience.
- Anticipated difficult intubation in uncooperative patient.
- Unanticipated difficult/failed intubation.

Contraindications

- Known or predicted difficulty in **mask ventilation**.
- Major bleeding in the upper airway.
- Upper airway obstruction.
- Risk of aspiration.
- Inexperienced anaesthetist.

- ## Teaching fibreoptic intubation in anaesthetized patients

The main indication for performing fibreoptic intubation in anaesthetized patients with normal airways is for teaching and training purposes. This training is useful before performing fibreoptic intubation on patients with a difficult airway.

Advantages

- Uninhibited conversation between the trainee and trainer.
- Controlled environment.
- Less time is needed than awake intubation.
- Anaesthetized patient has no discomfort.
- More patients are available than those requiring awake fibreoptic intubation.

Objectives

- Gain proficiency in fibreoptic endoscopy technique.
- Learn tracheal tube selection and railroading techniques.
- Learn fibreoptic techniques using airway aids.
- Learn principles of fibreoptic intubation under general anaesthesia in difficult airway patients.

Flexible fibreoptic-guided tracheal intubation is a three-stage procedure. The first, of fibreoptic endoscopy, guides the tip of the fibrescope into the trachea under continuous vision; the second, of railroading the tracheal tube over the insertion cord; the third, of checking tube position and removing the fibrescope from it. Achieving proficiency in fibreoptic endoscopy is vital and not only increases speed but also skill. During a nasotracheal endoscopy, trainees are encouraged to demonstrate anatomy through the nose (nasendoscopy), pharynx (pharyngoscopy), larynx (laryngoscopy) and trachea (tracheoscopy) in a sequential, unhurried manner by appropriate manipulations of the fibrescope. This technique avoids repetitive abrasion of the mucosal wall by the fibrescope and prepares the trainee to recognize abnormal anatomy, ensuring a high success rate in difficult airway patients. It is superior to the semi-blind techniques of either inserting the fibrescope directly in the nose or mouth, or by inserting it through a tracheal tube already inserted in the nasopharynx (tube-first method) and then wiggling its tip to find the glottis. Trainees also appreciate the difficulties caused by blood, secretions and airway collapse due to general anaesthesia and learn how to deal with them (see Chapter 10).

The second stage includes selecting appropriate tracheal tubes and learning the correct techniques of railroading them. Although the two stages are separately discussed, in practice they can be taught simultaneously.

Another important objective of learning fibreoptic intubation in anaesthetized patients with normal airways is to practise techniques using fibreoptic airway aids. Examples include various conduit airways for orotracheal intubation and fibreoptic-assisted intubation through the LMA (see Chapter 4). The possible application of these techniques in various clinical scenarios in patients with difficult airways (anticipated and unanticipated) is discussed in Chapter 5. The practical aspects of some of the scenarios are discussed later in this chapter.

● Upper airway anatomy through the fibrescope

It is essential to understand the upper airway anatomy as it is seen through the eyepiece of the fibrescope or on the monitor screen before attempting fibreoptic intubation in anaesthetized patients. This is best achieved by watching an instruction video or an experienced endoscopist demonstrating it on an anaesthetized patient. It must be appreciated that the appearances on the visual field are different, depending on whether the endoscopist is standing behind or in front of the patient.

Nasotracheal fibreoptic endoscopy

Endoscopist standing behind the head of a supine patient

Nose

The nose is one of the narrowest part of the upper airway and has an external opening (external nares or nostrils), nasal cavity and posterior openings (choanae).

Nostril

The tip of the fibrescope is inserted just inside the nostril. The more patent nostril is selected by direct inspection (Figure 6.1a). In this example, the right nostril is selected.

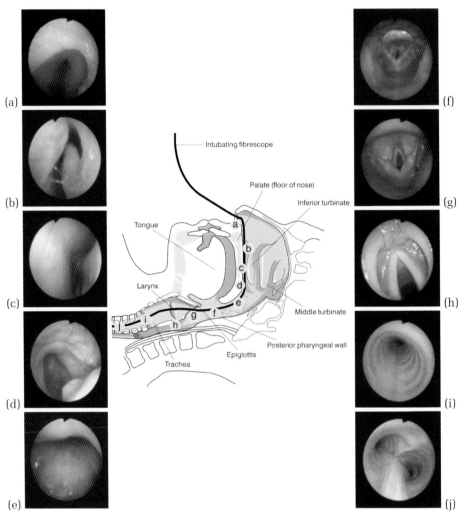

Figure 6.1 (centre) Upper airway anatomy during nasotracheal fibreoptic endoscopy. Endoscopist standing behind a supine patient. (a) The right nostril is selected. (b) The tip of the fibrescope is advanced in the triangular space bounded by the nasal septum (left) inferior turbinate (bottom) and lateral wall of the nose (right) of the visual field. (c) The fibrescope tip above the inferior turbinate which is to the right of the visual field. (d) The posterior opening of the nasal cavity is indicated by disappearance of inferior turbinate (at the 5 o'clock) position. The posterior pharyngeal wall is seen in the centre of the visual field. (e) The soft palate is seen in the upper part and the base of the tongue in the lower part. (f) Epiglottis in view. (g) Laryngeal inlet with vocal folds, vocal cords, cuneiform and corniculate cartilages. (h) True and false vocal cords. The posterior part of the glottis has a bigger airspace. (i) Trachea with tracheal rings. (j) Carina with openings of right and left main bronchi

Nasal cavity

A slight advancement of the tip in the neutral position brings the nasal cavity in view. The most important structures to identify are the nasal septum, inferior turbinate and the floor of the nose. It is important to understand that the floor of the nose appears on the top half of the monitor when the endoscopist stands behind a supine patient. In Figure 6.1(b) the nasal septum is on the left, the inferior turbinate on the bottom and the lateral wall of the nose on the right of the visual field. The tip of the fibrescope should lie in the triangular airspace bounded by these three structures (the airspace appears dark in the visual field). The journey through the rest of the nasal cavity is easy once the triangular airspace is found. The fibrescope tip is advanced towards the nasopharynx in this airspace which generally gets bigger (Figure 6.1c). A slight rotation movement will keep the airspace in the middle of the visual field. An unnecessary common mistake is to perform vigorous deflection of the tip in the nasal cavity.

Nasopharynx (posterior opening of the nose)

The beginning of the posterior opening of the nose is identified by the disappearance of the inferior turbinate. In Figure 6.1(d) it is seen just disappearing in the visual field at about the 5 o'clock position. The tip then enters the nasopharynx where the posterior pharyngeal wall is seen. In Figure 6.1(d) this is in the centre of the visual field. The tip is deflected slightly anteriorly to avoid contact with the posterior pharyngeal wall. A rotational movement will help to keep the tip of the fibrescope in the centre of the visual field and further advancement will bring it to the oropharynx.

Oropharynx

The soft palate (and sometimes uvula) is seen in the upper part, the posterior pharyngeal wall and base of the tongue in the lower part of the visual field (Figure 6.1e). The airspace may be collapsed due to general anaesthesia and a jaw thrust is required to open the airspace. The epiglottis immediately comes into view and is usually seen at a distance (Figure 6.1f). The fibrescope tip is then advanced towards the epiglottis, keeping its tip in the centre of the visual field.

Larynx

The tip of the fibrescope is deflected slightly posteriorly in order to pass it underneath the epiglottis when the vocal cords come into view (Figure 6.1g). Usually a full view of the laryngeal inlet is seen with the vocal cords, anterior commissure, vocal folds with the false cords, and cuneiform and corniculate cartilages. The posterior part of the glottis has a bigger airspace, and a slight posterior tip deflection will let it pass through the cords without touching them and into the trachea (Figure 6.1h).

Trachea and carina

The insertion cord is advanced into the trachea and the tracheal rings come into view (Figure 6.1i). The tip should stay in the lumen of the trachea without touching the walls. Further advancement will bring the carina in view (Figure 6.1j).

Orotracheal fibreoptic endoscopy

During orotracheal fibreoptic endoscopy, the fibrescope has to be manipulated in a bigger airspace and the angle at which the tip of the fibrescope hits the glottis is very acute. It is usual to use a conduit airway, e.g. Berman, for orotracheal fibreoptic intubation and the endoscopic pictures through a Berman airway are shown later, in Figure 6.8. The following is a description of the oropharyngeal anatomy as seen in the eyepiece or monitor screen without using a conduit airway.

Orotracheal fibreoptic endoscopy

Endoscopist standing behind a supine patient

The mouth and oral cavity

The fibrescope tip is brought near the mouth (Figure 6.2a). The mouth is opened and the tongue is seen on the top half of the monitor screen and the hard palate on the lower half (Figure 6.2b). The fibrescope tip is advanced in the midline. The airspace in a paralysed patient may be collapsed (Figure 6.2c). A jaw thrust manoeuvre or tongue traction opens up the airspace and the epiglottis is seen in the distance when the tip is slightly deflected anteriorly (Figure 6.2d). The tip is advanced further

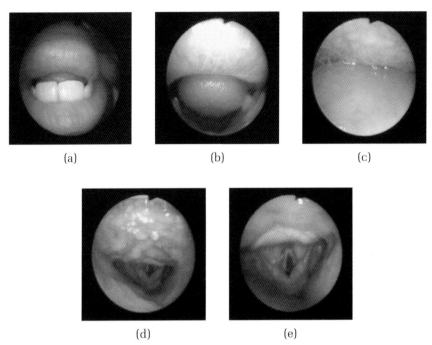

(a) (b) (c)

(d) (e)

Figure 6.2 Upper airway anatomy during orotracheal fibreoptic endoscopy – endoscopist standing behind a supine patient: (a) the fibrescope is brought near the oral cavity; (b) the oral cavity – the tongue is in the upper part and the hard palate in the lower half of the visual field; (c) in a paralysed patient the airspace may be collapsed; (d) jaw thrust or tongue traction opens the airspace and anterior deflection of the fibrescope tip reveals the epiglottis; (e) the fibrescope is advanced and the vocal cords are seen

and the vocal cords come into view (Figure 6.2e). From this point the description of the anatomy is the same as that described for nasotracheal endoscopy.

● Tracheal tube selection for fibreoptic intubation

Fibreoptic-guided tracheal intubation involves three separate stages:

- Successfully manipulating the tip of the fibrescope into the trachea.
- Railroading the tracheal tube over the fibrescope.
- Removing the fibrescope from the tube.

If a proper tracheal tube has not been selected, difficulty or even failure in railroading it may result, despite the tip of the fibrescope being in the trachea. This is due to the tip of the tracheal tube impinging on anatomical structures, usually the arytenoids, during its passage into the trachea. The success rate of intubation is high when attention is paid to detail in tracheal tube selection. Several factors influence this choice and include:

- The size of the tracheal tube.
- The flexibility of the tube and its tip design.
- The technique of railroading.

Whichever tube is chosen, railroading is facilitated when the insertion cord of the fibrescope is lubricated before loading the tracheal tube over it. A small piece of tape should hold it in place. It is important not to lubricate the outside of the tube to avoid it becoming slippery. The airspace must be open, if required by applying jaw thrust during railroading.

Size of tracheal tube

The larger the difference between the diameters of the fibrescope and tracheal tube, the greater is the difficulty in passing the tube through the cords. The grip for railroading is lost and the weight of the tube tends to make its tip impinge on the right arytenoid cartilage. When using an adult intubating fibrescope, 6–7 mm ID tracheal tubes are satisfactory. A study found 95% success rate with 6 mm tubes compared to 55% with 8 mm tubes for orotracheal fibreoptic intubation [1].

Flexibility and design of tracheal tubes

The flexibility of armoured (flexometallic) tubes conforms best to the fibrescope and results in a high first-pass success of 95% when compared with the 35% of rigid standard tubes [2].

The design of the tip of the tracheal tube influences the success rate of railroading (Figure 6.3). A newly designed tube with a conical, tapered tip without a bevel was superior to a standard tube during both oral and nasal railroading [3]. This tube is not available commercially. The dedicated intubating laryngeal mask airway tube is made of silicone and has a tapered tip. It has been shown to make intubation easier and faster when compared with a standard tube [4].

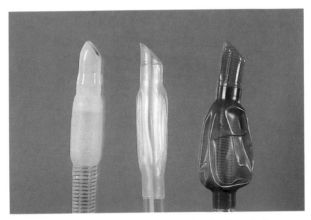

Figure 6.3   The flexibility and design of tracheal tubes influences railroading. The dedicated intubating LMA tube (left) and flexometallic tube (right) are better suited for railroading than a standard tube (middle)

Technique of railroading

Hold-up of the tracheal tube can occur due to the resistance of the laryngeal structures if the tracheal tube is advanced in the neutral position (with the tip of the tube to the right side and the bevel facing the left side). The right arytenoid is the commonest site for the tube to 'hang up' on when being threaded over the fibrescope [5]. A slight withdrawal and 90° counterclockwise rotation of the tube brings the tip of the tube to the 12 o'clock position and the bevel to the 6 o'clock position, permitting the tube to enter the trachea without resistance [6]. A clear airway must also be maintained by mandibular displacement (jaw thrust) while attempting to railroad the tube. A technique of continuously rotating the tube between the fingers while advancing it over the fibrescope has been described for flexometallic tubes [7].

My preference for nasotracheal intubation is to use preformed north-facing RAE tubes, 6–7 mm ID and warm them before loading onto the fibrescope. For orotracheal intubation, I use 6–7 mm south-facing oral RAE tubes or flexometallic tubes.

● Techniques of teaching fibreoptic intubation in anaesthetized patients

The essential requirements of a safe and effective technique are as follows:

- The patient should be anaesthetized at all times (avoid awareness).
- The patient should be adequately oxygenated and maintain an unobstructed airway at all times.
- Laryngeal reflexes should be obtunded with muscle relaxation or local anaesthesia.

Two primary techniques are possible, one in which the patient is paralysed, the 'apnoeic' technique, and the other in which the patient is breathing spontaneously, the 'spontaneously breathing' technique.

Apnoeic technique

This technique has been used in several studies for teaching fibreoptic intubation by the orotracheal [8–10] or nasotracheal route [11]. After intravenous induction, muscle paralysis is achieved with suxamethonium [9,12] or with a non-depolarizing agent, vecuronium or atracurium [8,9,11], while anaesthesia is maintained with an inhalation agent [11] or total intravenous anaesthesia [10]. The trainee performs nasal or oral endoscopy and intubation while the patient is 'apnoeic'. The period of apnoea is usually limited to 2–3 min. If the trainee fails within this time limit, or if oxygen saturation drops to less than 95%, manual ventilation is re-established and the procedure is repeated, usually once more [8]. If they are unsuccessful, the trainer performs the intubation.

Safety and effectiveness of the 'apnoeic' technique

Several workers have shown the safety and effectiveness of teaching fibreoptic intubation in anaesthetized paralysed patients [9–11]. The conditions are controlled with no coughing or laryngeal spasm. All the studies have shown that the time taken for fibreoptic intubation is longer when compared with conventional laryngoscopy. This raises the question of a potential for hypoxaemia and hypercarbia. This is prevented by limiting the intubation time to a maximum of 3 min after pre-oxygenation with 100% oxygen, mild hyperventilation, and stopping and re-ventilation with 100% oxygen if arterial saturation falls below 95% [9]. Because of the longer duration of fibreoptic intubation, the haemodynamic responses to fibreoptic intubation have been shown to be more severe than conventional intubation when using an inhalation technique with enflurane [13] or isoflurane [14]. However these responses are not different when fentanyl [15] or alfentanil [16] are included in an inhalation technique or if a total intravenous technique (TIVA) using propofol [17] is used. When fibreoptic and conventional laryngoscopy have been compared, no major differences have been found in the incidence of sore throat, dysphagia and hoarseness [8,10].

To overcome some of the limitations of the apnoeic technique and reduce the total apnoea time, a laryngeal mask airway (LMA) technique has been used during nasotracheal endoscopy teaching [18]. The LMA is inserted after induction of anaesthesia and muscle paralysis and the patient's lungs ventilated through it. The trainee performs a nasendoscopy in an unhurried fashion and when the tip of the fibrescope reaches the pharynx, the LMA is removed. Pharyngoscopy, laryngoscopy and tracheoscopy then proceed in the usual fashion. Osborne and colleagues were able to reduce the mean apnoea time to 59 s in the LMA group compared with 108 s in the group in whom no LMA was used. This technique is particularly useful for beginners when they are learning to perfect nasal endoscopy.

The apnoeic technique has been used to determine learning curves of proficiency in fibreoptic intubation. Most studies have suggested that trainees fulfil the objective of proficiency defined in the study by about the tenth intubation [8,9,19].

Spontaneously breathing technique

After intravenous induction, anaesthesia is maintained with inhalation anaesthesia or TIVA in a spontaneously breathing patient. Fibreoptic endoscopy is then performed by the nasopharyngeal or oropharyngeal route and, when the vocal cords are seen, intubation is performed under deep inhalation anaesthesia or after obtunding laryngeal reflexes with lignocaine sprayed through the working channel of the fibrescope. Oxygen can be delivered by nasal catheter or by using a fibreoptic airway aid, e.g. LMA [20], a chimney airway [21] capable of maintaining anaesthesia and oxygenation during fibreoptic intubation. A high incidence of laryngeal spasm, coughing and airway obstruction resulting in hypoxia have been reported when using this technique [22]. This study was, however, performed on patients with difficult airways and no pre-oxygenation was performed. This technique has the small advantage of 'creating' conditions that are seen during an awake fibreoptic intubation, i.e. spontaneous breathing, moving airway, spraying the cords.

Using these two primary techniques, various combinations of patient and anaesthetist positions are possible. These include keeping the patient supine or on the side with the operator standing behind the patient or on their side.

- ● **Teaching practical fibreoptic techniques under general anaesthesia**

Requirements

- ■ Experienced trainer.
- ■ Trainees (must have completed pre-clinical module).
- ■ Fibreoptic equipment with camera and monitor [11].
- ■ Trained assistant (for jaw thrust, preparing equipment).
- ■ Suitable patients (ASA I and II, normal airway, no risk of aspiration).

Steps of practical teaching technique 1 (Figure 6.4)

Nasotracheal fibreoptic intubation

Apnoeic patient in supine position

Anaesthetist standing behind patient's head

1. Check fibreoptic and anaesthetic equipment (see Chapter 1)
2. Commence standard anaesthetic monitoring.
3. Secure intravenous access.
4. Spray xylometazoline 0.1% (Otrivine®) drops into both nostrils for vasoconstriction.
5. Induce anaesthesia with fentanyl and propofol, muscle paralysis with vecuronium.
6. Institute manual ventilation with oxygen and isoflurane until muscle paralysis is achieved.
7. Anaesthetic assistant performs jaw thrust and assists trainee with fibreoptic equipment.
8. Trainee performs fibreoptic endoscopy while trainer monitors patient and guides trainee with the help of the fibreoptic camera monitor screen and times the endoscopy (Figure 6.5).
9. Trainee should show sequential nasal, pharyngeal, laryngeal and tracheal anatomy (see previous sections for diagrams).
10. If apnoea time exceeds 2 min or if oxygen saturation drops below 95%, re-establish ventilation with 100% oxygen.

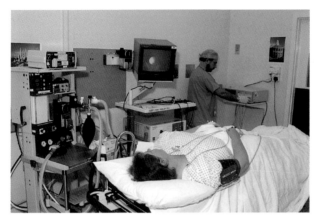

Figure 6.4   Anaesthetic room set up for teaching nasotracheal fibreoptic intubation in a supine patient. The anaesthetic, fibreoptic and monitoring equipment are checked and ready

11. Allow trainee a maximum of two attempts and if he/she is unsuccessful, trainer performs intubation with a fibrescope or conventional laryngoscope.
12. Railroad a 6–7 mm cuffed nasal RAE tracheal tube (previously warmed in sterile normal saline and loaded over the fibrescope) when the tip of the fibrescope has reached to

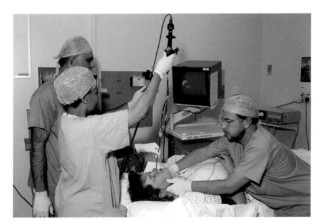

Figure 6.5   Teaching nasotracheal fibreoptic intubation in an apnoeic supine patient. The trainee performs nasotracheal endoscopy and the trainer guides her with the help of an endoscopic camera monitor system. The anaesthetic assistant provides jaw thrust

within 25 mm (1 in) of the carina. Rotate the tube 90° counterclockwise to bring the tip anteriorly.

13. Check the position of the tracheal tube by fibreoptic visualization, bilateral chest movement and presence of end tidal carbon dioxide.

Steps of practical teaching technique 2 (Figure 6.6)

Nasotracheal fibreoptic intubation

Spontaneously breathing patient, right lateral position

Anaesthetist standing on the right-hand side of patient and facing him/her

1. Check fibreoptic and anaesthetic equipment.
2. Commence standard anaesthetic monitoring.
3. Secure intravenous access.
4. Spray xylometazoline 0.1% (Otrivine®) drops into both nostrils for vasoconstriction.
5. Ask patient to lie on the right lateral side.
6. Induce anaesthesia with fentanyl, propofol and maintain with propofol infusion.
7. Administer oxygen through a suction catheter in one nostril.

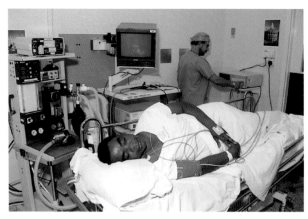

Figure 6.6 Anaesthetic room set up for teaching nasotracheal intubation in a spontaneously breathing patient lying on the right lateral side. The anaesthetic, fibreoptic and monitoring equipment are checked and ready. The patient is anaesthetized while lying on the side

8. Anaesthetic assistant assists trainee with fibreoptic equipment.
9. Trainee performs fibreoptic endoscopy while trainer monitors patient and guides trainee with the help of the fibreoptic camera monitor screen (Figure 6.7).
10. Once the vocal cords are visualized, obtund laryngeal reflexes with instillation of 4% lignocaine sprayed through the working channel of the fibrescope.

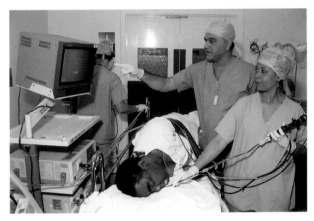

Figure 6.7 Teaching nastracheal fibreoptic intubation in a spontaneously breathing patient lying on the side. The trainee performs endoscopy while the trainer guides her with the help of endoscopic camera monitor system. Jaw thrust is usually not required

11. Railroad a 6–7 mm cuffed nasal RAE tracheal tube, previously warmed in sterile normal saline over the fibrescope when its tip has reached to within 25 mm of the carina. The tube is rotated 90° counterclockwise to bring its tip anteriorly.
12. Check the position of the tracheal tube by fibreoptic visualization, bilateral chest movement and presence of end tidal carbon dioxide.

● Teaching oral fibreoptic intubation in anaesthetized patients

Fibreoptic endoscopy via the orotracheal route is presumed to be more difficult than the nasotracheal route because:

- A larger airspace has to be negotiated in the oral cavity.
- The angle of attack from the oropharynx to the epiglottis is more acute.
- There is a tendency for the tongue to fall back and cause obstruction to the advancement of the fibrescope.

This problem is solved by asking an assistant to provide jaw thrust and tongue traction with an atraumatic tongue forceps [14] or by using a conduit airway, e.g. Ovassapian, Berman or bronchoscopy airway (see Chapter 4). These oropharyngeal airway aids act as a conduit for the fibrescope and help to keep its tip in the midline and prevent the tongue from obstructing the airway. The airway can be inserted either after full muscle paralysis or in the spontaneously breathing patient after inducing anaesthesia. The fibrescope is inserted through the lumen of the airway device, advanced through the larynx until the carina is seen, after which the tube is railroaded either with the airway device *in situ* or after it has been removed. Another method is to hold the fibrescope at a set distance with the thumb and index finger of one hand and then insert it in the midline while an assistant is providing jaw thrust [23]. This semi-blind method is not preferred in adults but may be useful in children (see Chapter 11).

Steps of practical teaching technique 3

> **Orotracheal fibreoptic intubation using Berman airway**
>
> **Apnoeic patient in supine position**
>
> **Anaesthetist standing behind patient's head**

Figure 6.8 illustrates the appearances of the visual field when orotracheal fibreoptic intubation is performed through a Berman airway (Figure 6.8a–d).

1. Check fibreoptic and anaesthetic equipment.
2. Commence standard anaesthetic monitoring.
3. Secure intravenous access.
4. Induce anaesthesia with fentanyl, propofol and muscle paralysis with vecuronium.
5. Manually ventilate the lungs with 100% oxygen and isoflurane until full muscle paralysis is achieved.

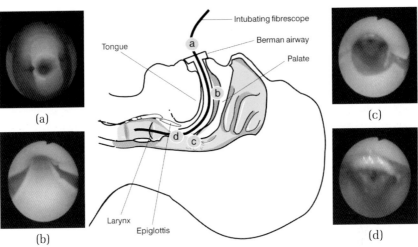

Figure 6.8 (centre) Endoscopic appearance during orotracheal endoscopy through a Berman Airway. (a) The tip of the fibrescope is inserted into the proximal opening of the airway. (b) Fibrescope tip in the lumen of the airway. (c) Fibrescope tip near the distal opening of the airway, showing slit opening on the right side. (d) Fibrescope out of the lumen of the airway. The upper flange is seen lifting the epiglottis

6. Insert a lubricated Berman airway in the oropharynx and confirm ventilation through it.
7. Anaesthetic assistant performs jaw thrust and assists trainee with fibreoptic equipment.
8. Trainee performs fibreoptic endoscopy by guiding the tip of the fibrescope through the Berman airway, under the epiglottis and through the vocal cords into the trachea until the carina is seen, while trainer monitors patient and guides trainee with the help of the fibreoptic camera monitor screen (Figure 6.9a).
9. If endoscopy time exceeds 2 min or if oxygen saturation drops below 95%, ventilate the lungs with 100% oxygen and isoflurane.
10. A maximum of two attempts are allowed for trainee and, if he/she is unsuccessful, then trainer performs the intubation.
11. A 6–7 mm cuffed oral tracheal tube, previously warmed in sterile normal saline, is railroaded over the fibrescope and through the airway when the tip of the fibrescope has reached to within 25 mm of the carina (Figure 6.9b).
12. Check the position of the tracheal tube by fibreoptic visualization, bilateral chest movement and presence of end tidal carbon dioxide.

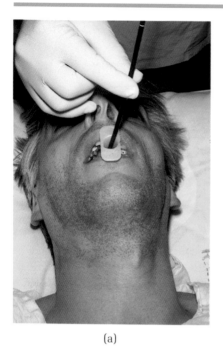

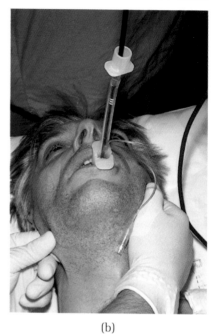

(a)

(b)

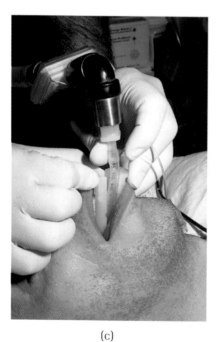

(c)

Figure 6.9 Orotracheal fibreoptic intubation through a Berman Airway: (a) the Berman Airway is inserted after induction of anaesthesia and muscle paralysis, and the intubating fibrescope is inserted through the lumen of the Berman Airway; (b) when the tip of the fibrescope is in the trachea, a cuffed tracheal tube is railroaded over the fibrescope; (c) the breathing system is connected and the Berman Airway is peeled off

13. Peel off the Berman airway from the tube or let it remain *in situ* (Figure 6.9c). Alternatively the Berman airway may be removed before railroading the tube. Any of the other conduit airways, such as an Ovassapian or a Bronchoscope airway, may be used instead of a Berman airway.

A technique of teaching orotracheal intubation with the patient on the side and the anaesthetist facing him/her is similar to the one that is described for this combination under nasotracheal intubation.

Teaching fibreoptic-assisted intubation through a LMA

The principles and techniques of fibreoptic-assisted intubation through a LMA have been discussed in detail in Chapter 4. This technique has an important role in intubating patients with a difficult airway (anticipated or unanticipated) under general anaesthesia (see Chapter 5). Teaching fibreoptic-assisted intubation through the LMA should be a priority in every training programme.

● Fibreoptic intubation under general anaesthesia in the difficult airway patient

This application of fibreoptic intubation in anaesthetized patients is discussed in Chapter 5. The clinical scenarios in which it has a possible role are summarized again as follows (see Table 5.2 for details):

■ Anticipated difficult airway but awake intubation not feasible.
■ Unanticipated difficult intubation during routine induction.
■ Unanticipated difficult intubation during rapid sequence induction.
■ Can't intubate, can't ventilate.

Anticipated difficult airway but awake intubation not feasible

In this clinical scenario, a patient with an anticipated difficult airway is unsuitable for an awake fibreoptic intubation usually because they may not cooperate during the procedure. Fibreoptic intubation under general anaesthesia is an option in these patients. Some practical points in the decision-making process are as follows:

- A thorough preoperative assessment of the airway is mandatory.
- The fact that an awake fibreoptic intubation would have been the technique of choice does not automatically mean that the patient should have fibreoptic intubation when they are anaesthetized. Other intubation options under general anaesthesia must be considered before a decision to perform fibreoptic intubation is made.
- However, the fibrescope is particularly useful in most cases where the problem is of difficult direct laryngoscopy due to anatomical features.
- It must be appreciated that the fibrescope is only an intubating tool and by itself does not provide any airway maintenance or ventilation. Before embarking to perform a fibreoptic intubation in these patients, one must ascertain that it is possible to keep the patient anaesthetized with an unobstructed airway and maintain oxygenation.

Once a decision has been made, the following practical points should be considered to achieve a high success rate without complications:

- Sedative premedication is desired, an antisialogogue is mandatory.
- Induction of anaesthesia can be by inhalation or intravenous route.
- Muscle paralysis should only be attempted if there is absolute certainty that manual ventilation is possible with a bag and mask.
- A technique using a conduit airway or LMA should be considered (see Chapter 4).
- A back-up plan (plan B) should always be worked out before embarking on the primary technique.

The role of fibreoptic intubation in the other difficult airway scenarios under general anaesthesia is discussed in Chapter 5.

● References

1. Koga K, Asai T, Latto IP, Vaughan RS. Effect of the size of a tracheal tube and the efficacy of the use of the laryngeal mask for fibrescope-aided tracheal intubation. *Anaesthesia* 1997; **52:** 131–5.
2. Brull SJ, Wiklund R, Ferris C, Connelly NR, Ehrenwerth J, Silverman DG. Facilitation of fiberoptic orotracheal intubation with a flexible tracheal tube. *Anaesth Analg* 1994; **78:** 746–8.

3. Jones HE, Pearce AC, Moore P. Fibreoptic intubation. Influence of tracheal tube design. *Anaesthesia* 1993; **48**: 672–4.
4. Lucas DN, Yentis SM. A comparison of the intubating laryngeal mask tracheal tube with a standard tracheal tube for fibreoptic intubation. *Anaesthesia* 2000; **55**: 358–61.
5. Schwartz D, Johnson C, Roberts JA. A maneuver to facilitate flexible fiberoptic intubation. *Anesthesiology* 1989; **71**: 470–71.
6. Hughes S, Smith JE. Nasotracheal tube placement over the fibreoptic laryngoscope. *Anaesthesia* 1996; **51**: 1026–8.
7. Calder I. When the endotracheal tube will not pass over the flexible fiberoptic bronchoscope. *Anesthesiology* 1992; **77**: 398.
8. Cole AFD, Mallon JS, Rolbin SH, Ananthanarayan C. Fiberoptic intubation using anesthetized, paralyzed, apneic patients. Results of a Resident Training Program. *Anesthesiology* 1996; **84**: 1101–6.
9. Johnson C, Roberts JT. Clinical competence in the performance of fiberoptic laryngoscopy and endotracheal intubation: a study of resident instruction. *J Clin Anesthesiol* 1989; **1**: 344–9.
10. Schaefer HG, Marsch SCU, Keller HL et al. Teaching fiberoptic intubation in anaesthetised patients. *Anaesthesia* 1994; **49**: 331–4.
11. Smith JE, Fenner SG, King MJ. Teaching fibreoptic nasotracheal intubation with and without closed circuit television. *Br J Anaesth* 1993; **71**: 206–11.
12. Roberts JT. Preparing to use the flexible fiber-optic laryngoscope. *J Clin Anesth* 1991; **3**: 64–75.
13. Finfer SR, Mackenzie JM Saddler, Watkins TG. Cardiovascular responses to tracheal intubation: a comparison of direct laryngoscopy and fibreoptic intubation. *Anaesth Intens Care* 1989; **17**: 44–8.
14. Smith JE, Mackenzie AA, and Scott Knight VCE. Comparison of two methods of fibrescope guided tracheal intubation. *Br J Anaesth* 1991; **66**: 546–50.
15. Smith JE, King MJ, Yanny HF et al. Effect of fentanyl on the circulatory responses to orotracheal fibreoptic intubation. *Anaesth* 1992; **47**: 20–23.
16. Hartley M, Morris S, Vaughan RS. Teaching fibreoptic intubation: effect of alfentanil on the haemodynamic response. *Anaesthesia* 1994; **49**: 335–7.
17. Schaefer H-G, Marsch SCU, Strebel SP, Drewe J. Cardiovascular effects of fibreoptic oral intubation: a comparison of a total intravenous and a balanced volatile technique. *Anaesthesia* 1992; **47**: 1034–6.
18. Osborn WA, Jackson AP, Smith JE. The laryngeal mask airway as an aid to training in fibreoptic nasotracheal endoscopy. *Anaesthesia* 1998; **53**: 1080–83.
19. Smith JE, Jackson APF, Hurdley J, Clifton PJM. Learning curves for fibreoptic nasotracheal intubation when using the endoscopic video camera. *Anaesthesia* 1997; **52**: 101–6.
20. Alexander R, Moore C. The laryngeal mask airway and training in nasotracheal intubation. *Anaesthesia* 1993; **48**: 350–51.
21. Coe PA, King TA, Towey RM. Teaching guided fibreoptic nasotracheal intubation. An assessment of an anaesthetic technique to aid training. *Anaesthesia* 1988; **43**: 410–13.
22. Smith M, Calder I, Crockard A, Isert P, Nicol ME. Oxygen saturation and cardiovascular changes during fibreoptic intubation under general anaesthesia. *Anaesthesia* 1992; **47**: 158–61.
23. Vaughan RS. Training in fibreoptic laryngoscopy. *Br J Anaesth* 1991; **66**: 538–40.

7

Awake fibreoptic intubation: general considerations

- Indications for awake fibreoptic intubation
- Contraindications for awake fibreoptic intubation
- Essential components for proper patient preparation
- Explanation and consent
- Premedication and premedication drugs
- Conscious sedation and drugs used for conscious sedation
- Monitoring
- Oxygenation
- Upper airway local anaesthesia
- Back-up plan if awake fibreoptic intubation fails

Flexible fibreoptic intubation is the technique of choice for securing airway patency while the patient is awake. A carefully planned technique that takes into account the patient's safety and comfort will ensure a high success rate. It is important to understand some essential components of the technique in order to achieve this goal. The principles of these components and their practical application are discussed in this chapter.

● Indications for awake fibreoptic intubation

The indications for performing awake fibreoptic intubation are summarized in Table 7.1. The causes of anticipated difficult intubation/mask ventilation and the role of awake fibreoptic intubation in its management are discussed in Chapter 5. A patient with a difficult airway and at risk of aspiration of gastric contents (trauma, emergency surgery and obstetrics) is safe when intubated awake. Methods of local anaesthesia in these patients are discussed in Chapter 8. Fibreoptic intubation performed

Table 7.1 Indications for awake fibreoptic intubation

Previous history of difficult intubation and/or mask ventilation
Anticipated difficult laryngoscopy on physical examination
Anticipated difficult mask ventilation
Risk of aspiration
Haemodynamic stability desired
Neurological assessment after intubation
Teaching, training and consolidation of experience

under topical anaesthesia is compatible with haemodynamic stability. It reduces the presser response to tracheal intubation in normotensive patients and is suitable for use in patients who are at risk from this response [1,2]. In many units, patients with an unstable cervical spine are assessed neurologically after intubation. Awake intubation is the technique of choice [3].

An important indication of performing awake fibreoptic intubation is for teaching, training and consolidation of experience. It is desirable that trainees gain supervised training in awake fibreoptic techniques before they perform them independently. A structured programme such as the one described in Chapter 2 is designed with this aim in mind. In most hospitals in the UK, an awake intubation is performed in only a small number of patients. A possible reason is a high threshold for performing awake intubation even in patients in whom difficulty is anticipated. Many patients in whom an awake intubation would be indicated are anaesthetized and intubated with suboptimal techniques, thereby compromising patient safety and denying the opportunity for consolidating experience and training.

Several approaches are possible to circumvent this problem. The first is to perform and teach awake fibreoptic intubation in all patients requiring intubation, so that the trainees learn these techniques from the start of their training. This approach has been used by Ovassapian in the USA, but is not popular in the UK [4]. It has obvious ethical and legal implications. A second approach is to send trainees to bronchoscopy clinics to learn topical anaesthesia and endoscopy techniques [5]. This may not be a possible arrangement in all departments. A third approach is to target operating lists where a high proportion of patients present with airway difficulties. We have successfully targeted a maxillofacial list where approximately 20% of patients have an awake fibreoptic intubation. With this approach the confidence of the trainer increases and the threshold for performing awake fibreoptic intubation decreases, thereby increasing the numbers suitable for training.

● Contraindications for awake fibreoptic intubation
(Table 7.2)

In most cases an awake fibreoptic intubation is an elective procedure and should be well planned. This includes getting help from an experienced anaesthetist if required. Awake fibreoptic intubation performed by an inexperienced anaesthetist will result in failure and can be psychologically damaging to the patient, who may then refuse the technique. The anaesthetist's morale will also be affected and he/she may get so upset by the events that they may never learn to perform fibreoptic intubation.

Table 7.2   Contraindications for awake fibreoptic intubation

Inexperienced anaesthetist
Patient refusal
Local anaesthetic sensitivity
Uncooperative adults
Most children
Massive haemorrhage in the mouth

Most patients will agree to the procedure if a proper pre-operative explanation of the technique, as described below, is given. If the patient still refuses, the alternative methods of airway control will have to be planned.

Local anaesthetic allergy is uncommon, but when present represents a contraindication to awake fibreoptic intubation.

Awake fibreoptic intubation is desirable but not practicable in some uncooperative adults; for example, patients with learning difficulties, language barriers and who have altered conscious level. Most children also fall under this category. Adequate sedation and topical anaesthesia are difficult to achieve in these patients and fibreoptic intubation under general anaesthesia (see Chapter 6) may be considered.

Massive haemorrhage in the oral cavity will interfere with the endoscopic view and is a relative contraindication. A larger diameter fibrescope with a bigger suction channel may successfully be used in some cases.

● Essential components for proper patient preparation

The essential components for proper preparation of a patient for awake fibreoptic intubation are shown in Table 7.3. Awake fibreoptic intubation is stressful for most anaesthetists and can be unpleasant and uncomfortable to the patient if they are not properly prepared. It is assumed that fibreoptic equipment and skilled assistance are available and the anaesthetist performing the technique is experienced.

Table 7.3   Essential components for proper preparation of a patient for awake fibreoptic intubation

Explanation and consent
Premedication
Conscious sedation
Monitoring
Oxygenation
Upper airway local anaesthesia
Back-up plan

● Explanation and consent

The history and examination of previous records and/or physical examination should confirm that the patient needs an awake fibreoptic intubation. A thorough, unhurried explanation of the technique should then follow. I explain to the patient why intubation is indicated and how this is usually performed in a patient with a normal airway. Then I explain the difficulties if intubation were performed after induction of anaesthesia and the safety of an awake fibreoptic technique. The patient is reassured that sedation would be provided for amnesia and comfort. The local anaesthetic technique is explained carefully and the patient is warned that this would take away the discomfort of the procedure but not provide complete numbness. It is easy to liken the procedure to an upper gastrointestinal endoscopy (with which a lot of patients are familiar), emphasizing that the intubating fibrescope is a much thinner tube but also explaining that railroading the tube may sometimes be uncomfortable. The patients are reassured that they will have a general anaesthetic once the tracheal tube is in place. This conversation acts as a way of explanation of the procedure, but more importantly establishes rapport with the patient.

Formal consent for the procedure always follows this discussion. Whether this consent is verbal or written depends on the local hospital policy. In our hospital we are not required to ask the patient to sign a consent form for the anaesthetic as long as we document the discussion in the notes. It is best for trainees to visit the patients with their trainers on the first few occasions. With experience and confidence their ability to communicate effectively with patients increases.

● Premedication and premedication drugs

The objectives of pharmacological premedication are to reduce anxiety and produce a dry mouth. Pharmacological methods of reducing anxiety are not a substitute for the psychological preparation mentioned above. Depending on the risk, prophylaxis for aspiration is also prescribed.

Sedatives and anxyolytics

Benzodiazepines

Benzodiazepines relieve anxiety and may produce amnesia. Any of the commonly used drugs such as temazepam, lorazepam or diazepam may be prescribed orally on the ward. Midazolam may be given intramuscularly, but its quick onset and short duration of action makes it ideal for intravenous administration in the anaesthetic room.

Opioids

Opioids such as morphine and pethidine do not relieve anxiety, but are mild sedatives and good analgesics. By administering morphine 0.1–0.15 mg/kg intramuscularly 1 h preoperatively, the need for additional intravenous opioids during the procedure is reduced, thus preventing airway obstruction and respiratory depression. Opioids may also aid endoscopy by depressing airway reflexes and suppressing cough. They may, however, cause nausea and vomiting and must not be administered to patients in whom there is a risk of airway obstruction.

Prophylaxis for aspiration

Some patients (e.g. obstetric, trauma, obese, history of reflux) undergoing awake fibreoptic intubation may be at risk of aspiration of gastric contents. A combination of an H_2 blocker (e.g. ranitidine 150 mg orally) to reduce the amount of acid in the stomach and metoclopramide 10 mg orally, a dopamine antagonist for stimulating the motility of the upper gastrointestinal tract, increasing the lower oesophageal sphincter tone and preventing vomiting, is the usual choice.

Antisialogogues

Antisialogogues should be administered before awake fibreoptic intubation for several reasons. A dry mouth ensures better contact between the local anaesthetic and mucosa, ensuring better absorption and longer duration of action of local anaesthetic [6]. Without antisialogogue pretreatment, local anaesthetic is diluted by saliva, decreasing contact with the mucosa and increasing the amount swallowed. Secretions may interfere with fibreoptic endoscopy; thick secretions may clog the working channel of the fibrescope; thin secretions may cause internal reflection and distort the view.

Anticholinergic drugs such as atropine, hyoscine and glycopyrrolate are effective antisialogogues. Atropine is best avoided because it is a weak antisialogogue and may cause tachycardia. Hyoscine may be given orally (0.4 mg) or intramuscularly (0.2 mg) 1 h preoperatively. It is a powerful antisialogogue and also produces sedation and amnesia. It is best avoided in patients over 60 years of age as it may cause confusion and disorientation. Glycopyrrolate is a quaternary ammonium compound and does not cross the blood brain barrier. It has a moderate antisialogogue effect and produces no sedation. It may be given intramuscularly (0.2 mg) or intravenously (0.2 mg), when its action starts in about 3 min. My preference is to give hyoscine 0.2 mg IM 1 h before endoscopy to patients under 60 years and glycopyrrolate 0.2 mg IM to patients over 60. If for some reason it is not possible to administer these drugs on the ward, 0.2 mg glycopyrrolate is given intravenously in the anaesthetic room as soon as intravenous access is secured.

● Conscious sedation and drugs used for conscious sedation

The term 'awake' intubation is a misnomer because, in practice, most patients receive some form of sedation during an 'awake' fibreoptic intubation. This is to relieve anxiety, produce amnesia and prevent discomfort or pain. Conscious sedation (CS) is a state where the patient can tolerate potentially unpleasant procedures without compromising cardiopulmonary function or the ability to react purposely to verbal commands and physical stimuli. It is not a substitute for a thorough explanation of the procedure at the preoperative visit. The characteristics of an ideal agent for CS are shown in Table 7.4.

Table 7.4 Characteristics of an ideal agent for conscious sedation

No pain on injection
Rapid onset of action
Short duration of action
Minimal cardiorespiratory depression
Easy to titrate dose to effect
Easy to administer as bolus or infusion
Availability of specific antagonist

Benzodiazepines

Benzodiazepines are good sedative, anxiolytic and amnesic drugs. They have no analgesic action.

Midazolam

This water-soluble benzodiazepine produces no pain on intravenous injection. It has a quick onset and short duration of action. Hypotension and respiratory depression are minimal when midazolam is given in small doses, but may occur with large doses and when the drug is combined with opioids, in the elderly and in patients with respiratory disease. Because of inter-patient variability in response, especially in elderly patients, over-zealous use may result in untoward sedation and respiratory depression.

Midazolam is contraindicated in patients with human immuno-deficiency disorders who are on protease inhibitors which may significantly alter the CNS effects of midazolam due to alteration of cytochrome P_{450} activity, resulting in increased plasma concentrations.

A common technique of providing CS is the use of intermittent boluses of midazolam and fentanyl. I prefer to dilute midazolam to 1 mg/ml (10 mg in 10 ml normal saline) and fentanyl 10 μg/ml (100 μg in 10 ml normal saline). Then boluses of 0.5–1 mg midazolam and 10–20 μg fentanyl are given, titrating the dose to effect. The effects of midazolam can quickly be reversed with a specific antagonist, flumazenil, should overdosage cause respiratory depression or airway obstruction. The initial dose is 10–20 μg/kg and can be repeated.

Diazepam

The injection is painful. Diazepam has a slower onset and prolonged duration of action. Midazolam has therefore largely replaced diazepam for the intravenous route.

Opioids

When given alone, opioids produce sedation but no anxiolysis or amnesia. They are powerful analgesics and suppress the cough reflex. Morphine has a slow onset and long duration of action, making it unsuitable for intravenous use during awake fibreoptic intubation. Drugs that are more lipid soluble and have a faster onset and shorter duration of action are commonly used intravenously.

Fentanyl

Fentanyl is a phenylpiperidine derivative and is 100 times more potent than morphine. It has a quick onset and short duration of action due to redistribution in inactive tissues such as fat and muscle. Unlike morphine, fentanyl does not produce histamine release, thus reducing the risk of hypotension. Chest tightness may occur with rapid injection. It may cause respiratory depression and drowsiness, especially when combined with midazolam. My practice is to dilute fentanyl to 10 μg/ml and give 1–2 ml at a time. Intravenous fentanyl is usually not required during the procedure if intramuscular morphine has been administered as a premedication.

Alfentanil

Alfentanil is 10 times weaker than fentanyl but has a slightly faster onset of action. It may be diluted to 100 µg/ml and given as boluses of 1–2 ml at a time.

Remifentanil

Remifentanil may have some advantages over the fentanyl congeners in providing the opioid component of sedation and analgesia for CS. Because of the ester structure, it is susceptible to ester hydrolysis, resulting in rapid metabolism. Its effects dissipate very quickly after an infusion is stopped. It has a very rapid onset, rendering titration of the infusion precisely controllable. Changes in the administration rate are quickly reflected in the level of drug effect. If an opioid effect is desirable, it can quickly be achieved with an increase in infusion rate. If toxic effects such as decreased respiratory rate or apnoea result, stopping the infusion will quickly reverse these effects. Infusion rates of between 0.05 and 0.175 µg/kg per minute have been used [7] for awake fibreoptic intubation.

Naloxone

Naloxone is a specific mu receptor antagonist. It reverses not only the respiratory depression but also the analgesic effects of opioids. It may also cause CNS excitation. I prefer to dilute naloxone to 40 µg/ml (400 µg in 10 ml normal saline) and give 1–2 ml at a time, titrating the dose to effect.

Propofol

Propofol is a phenol derivative that has been used as an anaesthetic since 1989. The painful intravenous injection can be prevented by prior injection of a small dose of lignocaine. Its advantages are a quick onset of action and rapid recovery due to redistribution from the central to the peripheral compartment. Propofol weakens the upper airway reflexes and is particularly suited to local anaesthetic techniques involving airway manipulation. It is easy to administer propofol with simple infusion pumps. The dose is variable and can be titrated between 0.5 and 2 mg/kg per hour. A simple and effective way of administering propofol by infusion is to give it on a mg/min basis regardless of patient weight and age, the usual dose being 1–2 mg/min. Target-controlled infusion (TCI) of propofol is also commonly used in anaesthesia. TCI propofol in a dosage range of 0.8–1.2 µg/ml has been used for CS during awake fibreoptic intubation [8]. The pump is simple and titration of propofol is easy in maintaining the desired sedation level and cardiorespiratory stability. Propofol does not provide amnesia and it may be necessary to administer a small dose of midazolam (0.5–1 mg) before commencing propofol infusion to ensure amnesia. Overdose with propofol may cause unconsciousness, respiratory depression and hypotension. There is no specific antidote available for reversing these effects.

Droperidol

Droperidol, a butyrophenol derivative, is an excellent sedative and when combined with fentanyl and midazolam produces a state of neurolept anaesthesia. It is also an antiemetic. Very small doses are effective. I prefer a dilution to 250 µg/ml (2.5 mg droperidol in 10 ml normal saline). Alternatively, 100 µg fentanyl and 2.5 mg of droperidol may be mixed in 10 ml normal saline in the same syringe and 1–2 ml of this mixture administered at a time, titrating the dose to effect.

Ketamine

Ketamine in a dose of 0.5–1 mg/kg is a sedative hypnotic. While the risk of airway obstruction and respiratory depression is low, there is an increased risk of salivation and hallucinations with its use. It is a useful agent in children (see Chapter 11).

● Monitoring

The level of consciousness should constantly be monitored to obtain the desired effect of the sedation regimen. The goal is a relaxed and calm patient who is able to respond appropriately to oral commands or mild physical stimuli. Over-sedation will lead to airway obstruction and cardiorespiratory depression, resulting in hypoxia. This may cause restlessness. On the other hand, under-sedation and inadequate local anaesthesia may also cause patient discomfort and restlessness. The depth of sedation must therefore be constantly monitored to determine the cause of the patient's restlessness and discomfort and take appropriate action.

Standard anaesthetic monitoring must be applied in the form of continuous ECG, pulse oximetry and intermittent blood pressure. A capnograph should be available to check the position of the tube when intubation is complete. If the general condition of the patient demands, other appropriate monitoring should be applied.

● Oxygenation

It is important to administer oxygen to the patient during CS. Hypoxia should be prevented by carefully titrating the sedation, but added oxygen will increase the reserves should it occur. During orotracheal fibreoptic intubation, oxygen is best delivered by nasal cannula. For nasotracheal fibreoptic intubation, I usually administer oxygen with an ordinary facemask while topical anaesthesia is being applied; after the nasal cavity is anaesthetized, a suction catheter is inserted in one of the nostrils and connected to the oxygen delivery tube. Many endoscopists prefer to deliver oxygen via the working channel of the fibrescope during endoscopy. This method has the advantage of not only delivering oxygen to the patient, but also pushes the secretions away from the tip of the fibrescope and helps in defogging the lens. Gastric distension and rupture has been reported with this technique [9].

● Upper airway local anaesthesia

Perhaps the most important component of the preparation of the patient for awake fibreoptic intubation is the achievement of perfect local anaesthesia of the upper respiratory tract. A meticulous technique allows this goal to be achieved, resulting in a comfortable patient who will then allow the anaesthetist to perform endoscopy and intubation in an unhurried manner. The final result is a very high success rate.

   The drugs used and the techniques of application of local anaesthetics to the upper airway are discussed in detail in Chapter 8.

● Back-up plan if awake fibreoptic intubation fails

It is essential that a back-up plan (plan B or C) is worked out in advance when planning management of a patient with a difficult airway. This will avoid complications and ensure patient safety in the event of failure of the primary technique. Awake fibreoptic intubation is a very safe technique with a high success rate, but difficulties and failures do occur occasionally. There are no hard and fast rules about back-up plans, but each case should be planned individually. The following options may be considered as back-up plans when awake fibreoptic intubation fails:

- Cancel the operation and regroup with more experienced staff.
- Proceed with surgical airway under local anaesthesia.
- Induction of general anaesthesia only, if mask ventilation is thought to be easy.
- Consider intubation options or surgical airway under general anaesthesia.
- Consider transtracheal jet ventilation before induction of general anaesthesia in difficult cases.

● References

1. Ovassapian A, Yelich SJ, Dykes HM, Brunner EA. Blood pressure and heart rate changes during awake fiberoptic nasotracheal intubation. *Anesth Analg* 1983; **62**: 951–4.
2. Hawkyard J, Morrison A, Doyle LA et al. Attenuating the hypertensive response to laryngoscopy and endotracheal intubation using awake fibreoptic intubation. *Acta Anaesthesiol Scand* 1992; **36**: 1–4.
3. Meschina A, Devitt JH, Koch JP, Schwartz ML. The safety of awake tracheal intubation in cervical spine injury. *Can J Anaesth* 1992; **39**: 114–17.
4. Ovassapian A, Yelich SJ, Dykes MHM, Golman ME. Learning fibreoptic intubation: use of simulators vs traditional teaching. *Br J Anaesth* 1988; **61**: 217–20.
5. Mason RA. Learning fibreoptic intubation: fundamental problems. *Anaesthesia* 1992; **47**: 729–31.
6. Watanabe H, Lindgren L, Rosenberg P, Randall T. Glycopyrronium prolongs topical anaesthesia of the oral mucosa and enhances absorption of lignocaine. *Br J Anaesth* 1993; **70**: 94–5.
7. Reusche MD, Talmage DE. Remifentanil for conscious sedation and analgesia during awake fibreoptic tracheal intubation: a case report with pharmacokinetic simulations. *J Clin Anesth* 1999; **11**: 64–8.
8. Kakodkar P, Lua S, Sear J, Popat M. Target controlled propofol for awake fibreoptic intubation. *Difficult Airway Society Abstracts*. Edinburgh 1999.
9. Hersley MD, Alexandar A, Hannenberg MD. Gastric distension and rupture from oxygen insufflation during fibreoptic intubation. *Anesthesiology* 1996; **85**: 1479–80.

8

Local anaesthesia for awake fibreoptic intubation

It is essential to understand the pharmacology of local anaesthetic drugs and the methods of their application in order to achieve effective local anaesthesia of the upper airway. When combined with appropriate sedation and a meticulous endoscopy technique, the highest degree of patient comfort and success rate are achieved.

Drugs used for local anaesthesia of upper airway

● Local anaesthetics

Local anaesthetics act by preventing depolarization of the nerve membranes that follows influx of sodium. Local anaesthetics are available as water-soluble acidic salts, and when injected or topically applied they are buffered in the tissues, releasing the free base. The free base is lipid soluble and penetrates the nerve tissue, producing anaesthesia. The release of the free base is delayed and the action of local anaesthetic is slow when the pH and buffering capacity of the tissues is lowered, as in infection. Topical local anaesthetics are less effective than injection techniques because of the low buffering capacity of the mucous membranes. A higher concentration of local anaesthetic is therefore required for topical anaesthesia. In the respiratory tract, the absorption of local anaesthetic is more rapid from the tracheobronchial tree than from the pharynx. Vasoconstrictors added to local anaesthetics for topical anaesthesia neither delay absorption nor prolong the duration of the action. Systemic effects of local anaesthetics are related to their plasma concentration. This depends on a variety of factors such as the total dose used, rate of absorption, distribution and metabolism. Metabolism is slow in patients with hepatic disease.

Cocaine

Cocaine is a natural alkaloid obtained from the leaves of *Erythroxylon coca*. It is the only local anaesthetic with vasoconstrictor properties. The vasoconstrictor properties are due to interference with reuptake of circulating catecholamines by the adrenergic nerve endings, the delay increasing catecholamine blood levels and producing vasoconstriction. Cocaine is an ester local anaesthetic, readily absorbed from the respiratory mucosa and slowly metabolized by pseudocholinesterase. Cocaine is generally available as 5% and 10% solutions, but other strengths are also available. It is a controlled drug. The 5% solution takes about 3–5 min to act, maximum plasma levels are reached in 60 min and metabolism takes 5–6 h. The 10% solution has a faster onset but may cause toxicity and should not be used. Signs of systemic toxicity include hypertension, tachycardia and cardiac arrhythmia. Body temperature may rise. The drug has powerful cortical stimulating action and may cause excitement, euphoria and increase in mental alertness. Cocaine in a dose of 2 mg/kg has been shown to cause coronary artery vasoconstriction, with a reduction in coronary blood flow and increased myocardial oxygen demands [1]. Cocaine should be used with caution in patients with hypertension, coronary artery disease [2], pre-eclampsia and with pseudocholinesterase deficiency. The maximum recommended dose of cocaine for topical anaesthesia of the nasal cavity is 1.5 mg/kg or 100 mg in a fit adult [3].

Lignocaine

Lignocaine is an amide local anaesthetic and is the most common drug used for local anaesthesia of the respiratory tract. It is a vasodilator and has a bitter taste. Many different preparations of lignocaine are available, such as aqueous 1%, 2% and 4% or viscous (gel) 2%, ointment 5%, 10% metered spray (10 mg per spray). The 4% solution is commonly used for topical anaesthesia of the upper airway and its action lasts for 15–20 min. The 2% solution is less effective but may be useful in children and for anaesthetizing the lower respiratory tract.

The rate of absorption of lignocaine depends on the surface area of the respiratory tract, the method of topical anaesthesia and whether the patient is breathing spontaneously or is anaesthetized and ventilated. Absorption of lignocaine is slower in the upper respiratory tract (oropharynx, nasopharynx, larynx) than the lower respiratory tract (bronchi, alveoli) because of its smaller surface area. A fraction of the lignocaine sprayed onto the oropharynx is removed during suctioning and some of it may be swallowed. About 70% of the swallowed lignocaine is metabolized in the liver at first pass. The plasma concentration of lignocaine is therefore lower with upper respiratory tract application than during lower respiratory tract application. Once in the plasma, lignocaine is metabolized by the hepatic micro-somal system. Lower doses of lignocaine should be used in patients with hepatic disease and low cardiac output states. In the conscious patient, toxic symptoms may appear with plasma levels of about 5 µg/ml [4]. The maximum recommended dose of lignocaine for topical application to the respiratory tract is 3 mg/kg [5]. In practice, higher doses, up to 9.3 mg/kg, have been used without systemic toxicity and peak plasma levels below the toxic levels described [6].

● Vasoconstrictors

The nasal mucosa is highly vascular and may bleed on instrumentation. Blood interferes with the fibreoptic view and may make a previously manageable airway impossible to intubate. It is therefore necessary to combine vasoconstriction when topical anaesthesia of the nasal mucosa is performed. Cocaine is both a local anaesthetic and vasoconstrictor, but some anaesthetists routinely avoid its use for fear of toxicity [7]. Its use is also contraindicated in certain conditions (see above). Other vasoconstrictors, usually mixed with lignocaine, may then be used to produce local anaesthesia and vasoconstriction.

Xylometazoline 0.1% (Otrivine®)

Xylometazoline is a sympathomimetic compound commonly used as a nasal decongestant in a spray form or as drops. It has been found to be as effective as cocaine in producing nasal vasoconstriction [8]. For topical anaesthesia of the nasal cavity, 5–10 drops (0.5 ml) are mixed with 4 ml of 4% lignocaine or 2% gel [7] to produce satisfactory anaesthesia and vasoconstriction.

Phenylephrine

Phenylephrine is an alpha agonist and a powerful vasoconstrictor. For topical anaesthesia and vasoconstriction of the nasal cavity, 4 ml of 4% lignocaine and 1 ml of 1% phenylephrine are mixed, resulting in a mixture of 3% lignocaine and 0.25% phenylephrine [9].

Methods of delivery of local anaesthetic to airway

Essentially there are three basic ways in which local anaesthetic can be applied onto the nerve endings:

1. Topical application of local anaesthetic.
2. Inhalation of nebulized lignocaine.
3. Nerve blocks.

● Topical application of local anaesthetic

Direct surface application of local anaesthetic on the mucous membranes of the respiratory tract is an easy and effective method. It is the most common of the methods used and is well tolerated by patients. There are several different techniques of applying local anaesthetics topically to the respiratory mucosa.

Direct application (with syringe or spray)

The local anaesthetic is applied on the mucosa with a syringe (Figure 8.1a) or spray. Examples are application of lignocaine gel

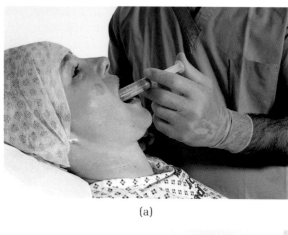

(a)

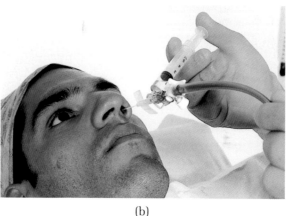

(b)

Figure 8.1 (a) Direct application of lignocaine gel to oral cavity. (b) Direct application of local anaesthetic using a 20 G Venflon catheter connected to oxygen tubing (green). The local anaesthetic blows in a jet when it is injected through the injection port with the oxygen flow at 2 litre/min

to the mouth or nose; 10% lignocaine spray to the back of the tongue and oropharynx. Another technique is to use a Venflon catheter connected to the oxygen tubing and applying the local anaesthetic from a syringe while the oxygen supply is running at 2 litres. This gives a jet-like effect and can be applied to the mouth or nasal cavity (Figure 8.1b) [10].

Application with ribbon gauze

This technique is useful for application of cocaine (or lignocaine and vasoconstrictor mixture) to the nasal cavity. A special ENT

Tilley forceps is used to pack the ribbon gauze into the nasal cavity (Figure 8.2a). The axis of the nasal cavity is perpendicular to the axis of the face, and local anaesthetic needs to be deposited in the airspace underneath the inferior turbinate along the floor of the nose. The angle of the Tilley forcep's directs the

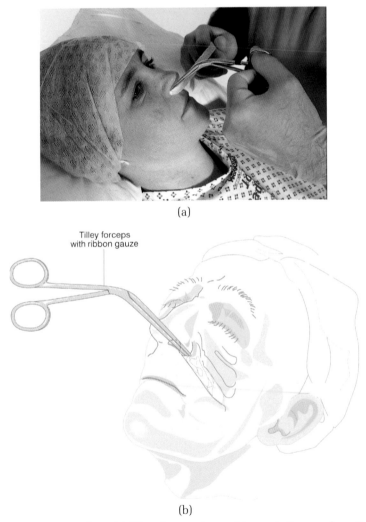

(a)

Tilley forceps
with ribbon gauze

(b)

Figure 8.2   A special ENT Tilley forceps is used to pack the nasal cavity with ribbon gauze dipped in local anaesthetic (a). The axis of the nasal cavity is perpendicular to the axis of the face. The angle of the Tilley forceps helps to deposit local anaesthetic underneath the inferior turbinade atraumatically (b)

ribbon gauze in this space atraumatically, thus avoiding bleeding and discomfort to the patient (Figure 8.2b). It is also possible to gauge the size of the nostril with this technique. Another advantage of this technique is that some of the cocaine is still soaked in the ribbon gauze when it is removed, thus reducing the amount of systemic absorption. I use a ribbon gauze of 30 cm length and 1 cm width soaked in 2 ml of 5% cocaine.

Cotton applicators

Cotton applicators mounted on sticks may be used instead of the ribbon gauze described above.

Spray as you go (SAYGO)

The working channel of the fibrescope can be used to instil local anaesthetic onto the mucous membrane of the respiratory tract. The technique must be performed carefully to prevent wastage of local anaesthetic and inadequate anaesthesia. The working channel of an intubating fibrescope (e.g. Olympus LF–2) is 600 mm long and 1.5 mm in diameter. If a small syringe is directly attached to the working channel port and the injection made, then it is likely to stay in the channel rather than be 'sprayed' onto the mucosa. Two adaptations to the technique avoid this problem (Figure 8.3a). First, 1.5–2.0 ml of 4% lignocaine are drawn up in 10 ml syringes and the plunger drawn right up so that the syringe contains a mixture of lignocaine and air. In this way, more force is created when the plunger is pressed down and the lignocaine emerges from the distal end of the working channel almost in the form of a jet. Second, a 16 G epidural catheter is fed through the working channel (distal end cut if a multi-holed catheter is used). The Luer-Lok connector of the epidural catheter gives a better grip to the syringe compared with the working channel port of the fibrescope, thus avoiding leakage of local anaesthetic. Additionally, when lignocaine is injected through the epidural catheter, an even larger force is created because the epidural catheter is narrower than the working channel of the fibrescope.

It is difficult for the endoscopist to perform SAYGO and keep the fibrescope in position. A trained assistant is therefore required (Figure 8.3b). The SAYGO technique can be quite unnerving to the novice because it causes coughing and each time the spray is performed the vision through the fibrescope

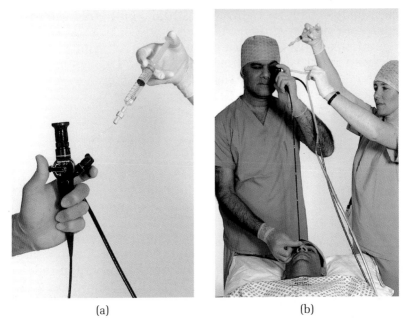

(a)   (b)

Figure 8.3 The SAYGO technique. Lignocaine 4% (1–2 ml) is drawn up in a 10 ml syringe and the plunger is fully drawn up. It is sprayed through a 16 G epidural catheter previously fed through the working channel of the fibrescope (a). It is difficult to perform SAYGO and endoscopy single-handed. A trained assistant performs SAYGO (b)

is lost. All that is required is patience, some suctioning of the local anaesthetic and deep breaths from the patient to get the view back.

● Inhalation of nebulized lignocaine

It is possible to anaesthetize the respiratory tract with lignocaine delivered through a nebulizer. Particles larger than 100 μm will concentrate in the oral mucosa, those between 60 and 100 μm in the trachea and main bronchi and those between 30 and 60 μm in the larger bronchi. In a nebulizer, 4–6 ml of 4% lignocaine is delivered in oxygen at a flow rate of 8 litres. The technique is easy to administer, safe, non-invasive and comfortable to the patient. Coughing is absent or minimal with this technique and therefore it may be useful in patients with increased intracranial pressure, open eye injury and unstable cervical spine injury.

Most anaesthetists feel that anaesthesia with this method is incomplete and requires additional SAYGO. It is also time consuming, almost taking 20–30 min, although good conditions have been reported in 5 min using 3 ml of 4% lignocaine and 1 ml of 1% phenylephrine [11].

● **Nerve blocks**

The nerve supply to the upper airway is derived from branches of cranial nerves V, VII, IX and X. Some of these nerves are suitable for blocking. To the anaesthetist performing their first awake fibreoptic intubation, it would appear that nerve blocks are an essential part of anaesthetizing the upper airway. This is not true and one learns that meticulous topical application is easier to perform, kinder to the patient and equally effective. Moreover, in some patients it is difficult or impossible to perform nerve blocks because of abnormal anatomy in the neck or upper airway. Techniques of two useful blocks, the glosso-pharyngeal and superior laryngeal nerve blocks, are described in this chapter. Although translaryngeal injection of local anaes-thetic through the cricothyroid membrane is regarded by some as recurrent laryngeal nerve block, it is not so (see below).

Techniques of upper airway anaesthesia

The following description is a systematic account of the different techniques, which may be used to achieve local anaesthesia of the upper airway (nasal cavity, oropharynx and larynx), for awake nasotracheal/orotracheal fibreoptic intubation. A sum-mary is shown in Table 8.1.

● **Nasal cavity**

Anatomy and nerve supply

The nasal cavity is innervated by a group of nerves from a variety of origins. The main supply is from the sphenopalatine ganglion, which receives branches from the gasserian ganglion via the trigeminal (V) nerve. Although other nerves are present, the greater and lesser palatine nerves provide sensory innervation of the nasal turbinates and to two-thirds of the posterior nasal septum. The anterior ethmoidal nerve, also a branch of the trigeminal nerve, gives sensory innervation to the anterior third of the nares.

Table 8.1 Summary of techniques of local anaesthesia for the upper airway

Anatomy	Nerve supply	Technique	Drugs
Nasal cavity	Trigeminal nerve	Topical-ribbon gauze or cotton applicators	2 ml 5% cocaine or 4 ml 4% lignocaine + 1 ml 1%phenylephrine
		Direct application	2% lignocine gel + 0.5 ml 01% xylometazoline
Tongue and oropharynx	Glossopharyngeal nerve	Topical gargle Topical spray Glossopharyngeal nerve block	2% lignocaine gel 10% lignocaine 2 ml 2% lignocaine
Larynx–supraglottic	Superior laryngeal nerve	Topical gargle SAYGO* Superior laryngeal nerve block	2% lignocaine gel 4% lignocaine 2 ml 2% lignocaine
Larynx–infraglottic	Recurrent laryngeal nerve	SAYGO* Translaryngeal injection	4% lignocaine 2 ml 4% lignocaine

*SAYGO = spray as you go through the working channel of the fibrescope.

Method of local anaesthesia

Topical application

Topical anaesthesia is the method of choice. It is simple to perform, very effective and is well tolerated by patients. Vasoconstriction is desirable.

Technique of topical anaesthesia

1. Patient sits up with anaesthetist facing him/her.
2. Introduce a length of fine ribbon gauze (1 cm wide) soaked with 2 ml of 5% cocaine in the airspace beneath the inferior turbinate with an ENT Tilley forceps (see Figure 8.2a).
3. Keep the ribbon gauze in the nasal cavity for about 5 min.
4. Alternatively, use cotton tip applicators or instil solution into nose with a syringe.

If cocaine is contraindicated or not desired, use 4 ml of 4% lignocaine solution or 2% gel [12] and add either 1 ml of 1% phenylephrine or 0.5 ml of xylometazoline for vasoconstriction.

● Tongue and oropharynx

Anatomy and nerve supply

The anterior two-thirds of the tongue receives sensory nerve supply from the trigeminal (V) nerve. The posterior one-third of the tongue and the oropharynx are supplied by a plexus from the facial (VII), glossopharyngeal (IX) and vagus (X) nerves. The lingual branch of the glossopharyngeal nerve supplies the sensory innervation to the vallecula, anterior surface of the epiglottis, posterior and lateral walls of the pharynx and tonsillar pillars.

Method of anaesthesia

Topical application

This is usually adequate, easy to perform and is well tolerated by the patient.

Technique of topical anaesthesia

1. Patient sits up with anaesthetist facing him/her.
2. Apply 4–6 ml of 2% lignocaine gel (Instillagel®) to the back of the tongue and ask patient to gargle it (see Figure 8.1a).
3. Patient may then spit the excess away or swallow it.

4. Apply the tip of a suction catheter to the oropharynx to check weakening of the gag reflex.
5. Apply more lignocaine gel if required.
6. Patients prefer lignocaine gel to the solution and it is easier to gargle [12].
7. A 10% lignocaine metered spray may be used instead of lignocaine gel.

Glossopharyngeal nerve block

The gag reflex arises from stimulation of deep pressure receptors found in the posterior one-third of the tongue. These receptors cannot easily be reached by diffusion of local anaesthetics through the mucosa. A glossopharyngeal nerve block is useful when it is desired to abolish the gag reflex completely.

An anterior approach – injection into the palatoglossal fold – or posterior approach – injection into the palatopharyngeal fold – can block the glossopharyngeal nerve (lingual branches). A bilateral injection blocks the sensory fibres (pharyngeal, lingual and tonsillar) and the motor branch to the stylopharyngeus muscles. The anterior approach is described below.

Glossopharyngeal nerve block – anterior approach

1. Patient sits up and anaesthetist faces him/her, standing on the contralateral side.
2. Ask patient to open the mouth as wide as possible and retract the tongue medially with a tongue depressor or gloved finger.
3. The base of the palatoglossal (anterior) arch forms a U- or J-shaped band of tissue, starting from the base of the palate, running along the lateral palatal wall to the lateral margin of the tongue (Figure 8.4a).
4. Use a 25 G spinal needle to inject 2 ml of 2% lignocaine at a point 0.5 cm from the lateral margin of the tongue at the point at which it joins the floor of the mouth (the trough of the 'U' or 'J') (Figure 8.4b) [13].
5. Perform an aspiration test. If air is aspirated, the needle is too deep, so withdraw it; if blood is aspirated, withdraw the needle and redirect medially.
6. Perform a similar injection on the other side.

Complications of glossopharyngeal nerve block

No major complications have been reported with the anterior approach, but accidental injection in the airway and blood vessels is possible. Haematoma, abscess and airway obstruction are potential risks of this block. With the posterior approach, headaches, seizures and dysrhythmias due to intravascular injection have been reported [14].

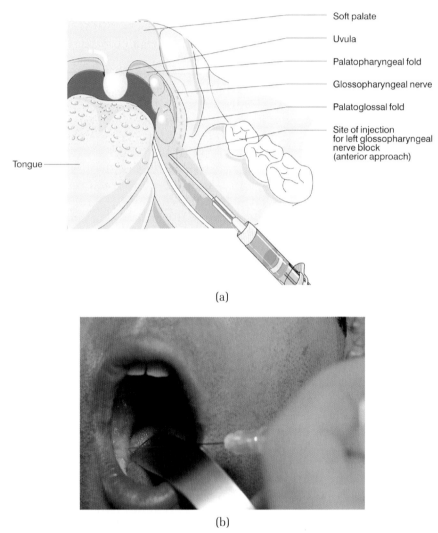

(a)

(b)

Figure 8.4 Glossopharyngeal nerve block – anterior approach: (a) the base of the palatoglossal arch forms a U- or J-shaped band of tissue, starting from the base of the palate and running along the lateral palatal wall to the lateral margin of tongue; (b) a 25 G spinal needle is used to inject local anaesthetic at a point 0.5 cm from the lateral margin of the tongue at a point where it joins the floor of the mouth (the trough of the 'U' or 'J')

● Larynx – supraglottic region (laryngeal inlet)

Anatomy and nerve supply (Figure 8.5)

The superior laryngeal nerve is a branch of the vagus (X) nerve arising from the inferior ganglion. It descends in the neck on the side of the pharynx deep to the internal carotid artery and divides into the external and internal laryngeal nerves. The

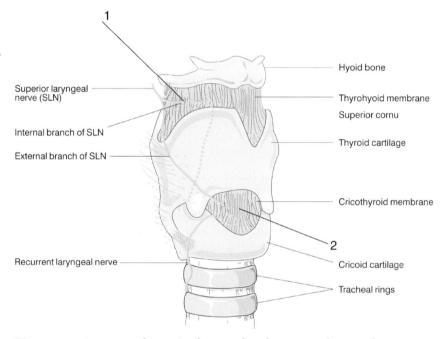

Figure 8.5 Anatomy of superior laryngeal and recurrent laryngeal nerves. 1 = injection site for superior laryngeal nerve block (external approach); 2 = injection site for translaryngeal injection (cricothyroid puncture)

former continues downward to supply the cricothyroid muscle and has no sensory distribution. The internal laryngeal nerve passes downward and forward to reach the thyroid membrane, which it pierces to enter the narrow space between the membrane in front and the epiglottis and pharyngeal mucosa behind. There it divides into its terminal branches that are sensory to the base of the tongue, vallecula, epiglottis, aryepiglottic folds, arytenoids and mucosa, down to but excluding the vocal cords.

Methods of local anaesthesia

Topical application

The patient sits up when topical anaesthesia to the nose and oropharynx (see above) is applied. By gravity, some of the gel will trickle onto the supraglottic region of the larynx. This is usually indicated by a slight cough. The anaesthesia is not always complete.

Spray as you go (SAYGO)

The technique of SAYGO has been described above. The spraying should start as soon as the epiglottis comes into view. Normally 2–3 sprays of 1.5–2 ml of lignocaine 4% are required on the epiglottis and under it before the tip of the fibrescope enters the glottis. The vocal cords do not completely stop moving.

Superior laryngeal nerve block (SLNB)

The superior laryngeal nerve can be blocked by as many as three external and one internal (using Krause's forceps) approaches. One external method is described below. The injection is made through the thyrohyoid membrane in the space bounded by the membrane laterally and the laryngeal mucosa medially.

Technique of SLNB – external approach (Figure 8.6)

1. Patient sits up with anaesthetist facing him/her (on the same side of the block).
2. Identify the superior cornu of the hyoid bone beneath the angle of the mandible and in front of the carotid artery. It can be palpated with the thumb and index finger on the side of the neck as bilateral rounded structures.
3. Identify the superior cornu of the thyroid cartilage. It is recognized by palpating the thyroid notch (Adam's apple) and tracing the upper edge of the thyroid cartilage posteriorly when the superior cornu will be palpated as a small rounded structure lying just underneath the superior cornu of the hyoid bone on both sides.
4. Using a 4 cm, 25 G needle, walk along the superior cornu of the thyroid cartilage in a superior and anterior direction, aiming toward the lower third of the membrane.

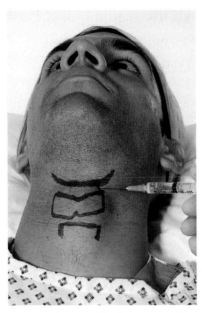

Figure 8.6 Superior laryngeal nerve block – external approach. Identify the superior cornu of the thyroid cartilage and direct the needle anteriorly and superiorly in the thyrohyoid membrane until a give is felt

5. When a give is felt, pierce the membrane and perform an aspiration test.
6. If air is aspirated, the needle is too deep and needs to be withdrawn.
7. If blood is aspirated, remove the needle and redirect it.
8. Inject 2 ml of 2% lignocaine with 1:200 000 adrenaline.
9. Perform a similar block on the other side.

Complications and precautions of SLNB

Accidental injection into the thyroid cartilage may paralyse the vocal cords, resulting in airway obstruction. Intravascular injection may cause hypotension and bradycardia and seizures. Pharyngeal puncture and haematoma are also possible risks of this block.

Contraindications for SLNB

Poor anatomical landmarks due to disease, local infection or local tumour growth. Not safe in patients with coagulopathy and those at risk of aspiration.

● Larynx – infraglottic region (vocal cords and trachea)

Anatomy and nerve supply (see Figure 8.7)

The sensory innervation of the vocal cords and trachea is supplied by the vagus nerve via the recurrent laryngeal nerves. The recurrent laryngeal nerves ascend along the tracheo-oesophageal groove and supply sensory fibres to the whole of the tracheobronchial tree, up to and including the vocal cords and motor supply, to all the intrinsic muscles of the larynx except the cricothyroid. The sensory and motor fibres run together. For this

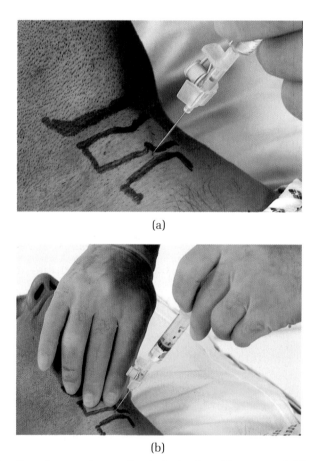

(a)

(b)

Figure 8.7 Translaryngeal anaesthesia (cricothyroid puncture). Identify the cricothyroid membrane as the space immediately below the inferior margin of thyroid cartilage with the patient supine and head extended (a). Stabilize the thyroid cartilage with the thumb and third digit of one hand and perform the injection with the other hand (b)

reason, recurrent laryngeal nerve blocks are not performed because this would result in bilateral vocal cord paralysis and airway obstruction.

Method of local anaesthesia

Spray as you go (SAYGO)

The vocal cords are sprayed and time given for the solution to work and patient to settle down. One or two sprays are performed once the tip of the fibrescope is in the trachea to anaesthetize the carina and reduce the intensity of coughing during railroading.

Translaryngeal anaesthesia (cricothyroid puncture)
(see Figure 8.7)

Technique of translaryngeal anaesthesia

1. Patient lies supine with the neck extended and anaesthetist standing to the side.
2. Identify the inferior margin of the thyroid cartilage. The space immediately below it and between the cricoid is the cricothyroid membrane (Figure 8.7a).
3. Make a small wheal of local anaesthetic intradermally.
4. With the thumb and third digit of one hand, stabilize the trachea by holding the thyroid cartilage (Figure 8.7b).
5. Remove the cap of a 20 G intravenous cannula (Venflon, Abbocath) and fix a 5 ml syringe containing 2 ml of 4% lignocaine to it.
6. With the other hand, insert the cannula so that its tip is facing caudad, always aspirating until a give is felt and air is aspirated.
7. Advance the cannula over the needle and then remove the syringe and needle from the cannula.
8. Reattach the syringe to the cannula and perform aspiration again to confirm the presence of the cannula in the airway.
9. Perform the injection at the end of normal expiration. This will ensure airway anaesthesia both below the vocal cords and up to the carina. The patient will cough during this procedure.

Cautions, complications and contraindications

The technique is safer when performed with a cannula. In 17 500 blocks, the only complications noted were two broken needles, two cases of severe laryngeal spasm and four cases of soft tissue infection [15]. More recently, a case of subcutaneous emphysema has been reported [16]. Studies during fibreoptic bronchoscopy suggest that translaryngeal anaesthesia produces the least coughing during endoscopy, but the most coughing during administration [17].

The block is relatively contraindicated in patients with raised intraocular and intracranial pressure, in patients with cervical spine injuries and in patients at risk of aspiration. It should not be performed in patients with bleeding tendencies.

● References

1. Lange RA, Cigarroa RG, Yancy Jr CW et al. Cocaine induced coronary vasoconstriction. *N Engl J Med* 1989; **321:** 1557–62.
2. Chiu CY, Brecht K, Dasgupta DS, Mhoon E. Myocardial infarction with topical cocaine anaesthesia for nasal surgery. *Archives of Otolaryngology – Head and Neck Surgery* 1986; **112:** 988–90.
3. Local anaesthetics – cocaine in *British National Formulary* March 2000; **39:** 576.
4. Foldes FF, Malloy R, McNall PG, Kaukal LR. Comparison of toxicity of intravascularly given local anaesthetic agents in man. *JAMA* 1969; **72:** 1493–8.
5. Shelley MP, Wilson JP, Norman J. Sedation for fibreoptic bronchoscopy. *Thorax* 1989; **44:** 769–75.
6. Efthimou J, Higenbottam T, Holt D, Cochrane GM. Plasma concentrations of lignocaine during fibreoptic bronchoscopy. *Thorax* 1982; **37:** 68–71.
7. Sidhu VS, Whitehead EM, Ainsworth QP et al. A technique of awake fibreoptic intubation: experience in patients with cervical spine disease. *Anaesthesia* 1993; **48:** 910–13.
8. Wright RG, Cochrane T. A comparison of the effects of two commonly used vasoconstrictors on nasal blood flow and nasal airflow. *Acta Otolaryngologica* 1990; **109:** 137–41.
9. Hartigan ML, Cleary JL, Gross JB, Schaffer DW. Is nasal cocaine superior to a lidocaine phenylephrine mixture for blind nasotracheal intubation. *Anesth Analg* 1984; **63:** 227.
10. Mackenzie I. A new method of drug application to the nasal passage. *Anaesthesia* 1998; **53:** 309–10.
11. Bourke DL, Katz J, Thonnsen A. Anesthesia for awake endotracheal intubation. *Anesthesiology* 1985; **63:** 690–92.
12. Webb AR, Woodhead MA, Dalton HR, Grigg JA, Millard FJC. Topical nasal anaesthesia for fibreoptic bronchoscopy: patients' preference for lignocaine gel. *Thorax* 1989; **44:** 674–5.
13. Benumof JL. Management of the difficult airway. *Anesthesiology* 1991; **75:** 1087–110.
14. Demeester TR, Skinner DB et al. Local nerve block anaesthesia for peroral endoscopy. *Ann Thorac Surg* 1977; **24:** 278.
15. Gold MI, Buechel DR. Translaryngeal anesthesia. A review. *Anesthesiology* 1959; **20:** 181–5.
16. Wong TW, McGuire GP. Subcutaneous emphysema following trans-cricohyroid membrane injection of local anaesthetic. *Can J Anesth* 2000; **47:** 165–8.
17. Graham DR, Hay JG, Clague J et al. Comparison of three different methods used to achieve local anesthesia for fibreoptic bronchoscopy. *Chest* 1992; **102:** 704–7.

9

Practical awake fibreoptic intubation techniques

The general principles of patient preparation and techniques of local anaesthesia for awake fibreoptic intubation are discussed in previous chapters. There are several ways to perform each aspect of awake fibreoptic intubation. Faced with these choices, one may ask if there is an 'ideal' technique. The simple answer is that there is not. Most anaesthetists start with a technique that they learnt from their first teacher and then fine-tune it. A good rule is not to practise a new technique each time.

It is easier to understand awake fibreoptic intubation techniques if the procedure is broken down into three stages as follows:

Stage one: Decisions
Stage two: Preparation
Stage three: Performing

Stage one: Decisions before awake fibreoptic intubation

The anaesthetist contemplating an awake fibreoptic intubation should make decisions about the following **before** the stages of 'preparing' and 'performing' (Table 9.1).

Table 9.1   Decisions for awake fibreoptic intubation

1. Choice of premedication
2. Sedation or no sedation
3. Operator and patient position
4. Local anaesthetic technique
5. Intubation route
6. Choice of tracheal tube
7. What is plan B?

Choice of premedication

Antisialogogue premedication is essential before every awake fibreoptic intubation. I prefer to give hyoscine 0.2 mg IM or glycopyrrolate 0.2 mg IM on the ward 1 h before the procedure. I also prefer to give morphine IM if there is no contraindication. Remember to prescribe aspiration prophylaxis if indicated.

Sedation or no sedation

Most patients will benefit from conscious sedation. Decide the drugs you want to use. Take extreme care when patients are at risk of respiratory depression, airway obstruction or aspiration.

Operator and patient position

The best position is one in which the patient is comfortable and the one that is most familiar to you. I prefer to sit up the patient during topical anaesthesia of the nasal and oral cavity. Once this is done, I perform the fibreoptic endoscopy standing behind the patient's head and with the patient in the supine position. I am prepared, however, to lay the patient on the side or sit them up if there is a good reason to do so; for example when there is risk of aspiration or airway obstruction.

Local anaesthetic technique

Nerve blocks are rarely required so do not worry if you are unable to perform them. Both translaryngeal injection and the SAYGO technique work well and are worth learning. With the translaryngeal injection technique, the patient coughs during the procedure but not so much during the endoscopy, so this is a good technique for beginners. The SAYGO technique causes more coughing and distortion of view but is suitable in most patients, even those with anatomical distortion of the airway and risk of aspiration.

Intubation route

The nasal route provides a more favourable angle for guiding the tip of the fibrescope to the laryngeal inlet. Topical anaesthesia is easy, and complete abolition of the gag reflex is not required. There is no danger of patients biting on the fibrescope and patients generally tolerate a nasal tube better while awake – a definite advantage at extubation. The disadvantages are the small risk of bleeding and discomfort during railroading. For these reasons some anaesthetists prefer to use the nasal route routinely unless there is a contraindication. Nasotracheal intubation is contraindicated in presence of nasal pathology such as fracture, bleeding, CSF leak or nasal surgery. I also avoid the nasal route in pregnant patients because of nasal congestion.

Choice of tracheal tube

It is easier to railroad a tracheal tube when the difference in diameter of the fibrescope (4 mm) and the internal diameter of the tracheal tube is small. Most patients can be adequately ventilated with small tubes [1] and tubes larger than 7.0 mm ID are rarely required. I use either preformed RAE or flexometallic tubes.

What is plan B?

A back-up plan must always be worked out **before** the procedure. Remember that this may involve getting help from a colleague or the surgeon and may require extra equipment.

In the examples that follow, the procedure has been broken into two further stages, preparing and performing, each with many steps to emphasize the details of each aspect of the technique. Paying attention to the minute details increases patient comfort and ensures a high success rate. In practice, most of the steps are performed simultaneously. Initially each step has to be thought through carefully and takes time, but with experience, awake fibreoptic intubation can be very rapidly and efficiently performed. I have given examples of only two techniques of awake fibreoptic intubation, one nasotracheal and one orotracheal, illustrating different techniques of sedation and local anaesthesia. In practice, one can use various combinations of these techniques to suit their practice.

● Example 1: Awake nasotracheal fibreoptic intubation

In the following example a decision has been made to perform an awake nasotracheal fibreoptic intubation with a nasal RAE tube. The SAYGO technique for local anaesthesia and midazolam/fentanyl boluses for sedation will be used. The anaesthetist will stand behind a supine patient.

Stage two: Preparing for awake nasotracheal fibreoptic intubation

The steps of this stage are summarized in Table 9.2.

Table 9.2   Preparing for awake fibreoptic intubation

1. Preparation in anaesthetic room
2. Preparation for local anaesthesia
3. Preparation for sedation
4. Preparation for intravenous induction
5. Preparation for back-up plan (plan B)

Preparation in anaesthetic room

- Check anaesthetic equipment.
- Check monitoring equipment.
- Check fibreoptic endoscopy equipment (see Chapter 1).
- Select tracheal tube: nasal RAE.

Preparation for local anaesthesia

All the equipment and drugs needed for local anaesthesia are arranged in a dedicated tray. Stocks are stored in the difficult airway trolley. This is convenient, saves time and ensures uniformity.

- Ribbon gauze (1 cm), cocaine 5%, Tilley forceps.
- 2% lignocaine gel (Instillagel®) 10 ml.
- Six 10 ml syringes filled with 1.5 ml of 4% lignocaine and air.
- 16 G epidural catheter threaded in the working channel of the fibrescope.

Preparation for sedation

- 10 mg midazolam diluted to 10 ml in normal saline.
- 100 µg fentanyl diluted to 10 ml in normal saline.

Preparation for intravenous induction

- Propofol or other induction agent.
- Muscle relaxant if appropriate.

Preparation for back-up plan if awake fibreoptic intubation fails

- Transtracheal jet ventilation equipment (if appropriate).
- Surgeon aware of need for tracheostomy (if appropriate).

Stage three: Performing awake nasotracheal fibreoptic intubation

The steps of this stage are listed in Table 9.3.

Table 9.3   Performing awake nasotracheal fibreoptic intubation

1. General
2. Preparing the nasal cavity and oropharynx
3. Final checks before endoscopy
4. Nasal endoscopy and SAYGO
5. Railroading the tracheal tube
6. Confirmation of tracheal tube position

General

1. Secure intravenous access.
2. Commence ECG and pulse oximetry monitoring and obtain blood pressure reading.
3. Sit up patient on the trolley at 60°.
4. Administer midazolam 0.5–1 mg bolus at a time until patient is relaxed but can still open eyes, move limbs and communicate verbally.
5. Administer supplemental oxygen with a facemask.

Preparing the nasal cavity and oropharynx

1. Apply ribbon gauze soaked with 2 ml of 5% cocaine into both nostrils with Tilley forceps with patient still sitting.
2. Instil 4–6 ml of 2% lignocaine gel to the back of the mouth. Ask patient to gargle the solution in the mouth. Warn them that the taste will be bitter.
3. After about 1 min, gently suck the back of the throat with a suction catheter to remove excess gel and to confirm that the gag reflex has weakened.
4. Instil 2–4 ml more gel if required.

Final checks before endoscopy

1. Remove the ribbon gauze from the nostril and ask patient to lie supine.
2. Select the best nostril by inspection under direct vision or with the fibrescope.
3. Continue administering oxygen with the suction catheter through the nostril that is not used for endoscopy.
4. Ensure once again that the suction tubing is attached to the fibrescope, the epidural catheter is in place and assistant knows how to inject through the scope.
5. Ensure that the tracheal tube is loaded onto the fibrescope.
6. Ensure patient is now supine and comfortable and administer more midazolam if required before endoscopy.

Nasal endoscopy and SAYGO

1. Standing behind the head of patient, commence nasendoscopy, identifying the inferior turbinate, and advance the tip of the fibrescope in the space underneath it. (The inferior turbinate is seen on the lateral side and the space appears on

the top of the monitor screen in this position – see Chapter 6.) Advance the fibrescope and keep the tip of the fibrescope in the centre of the visual field in the airspace.

2. On entering the oropharynx, help may be required from the patient to open the airspace by asking him/her to take deep breaths or stick the tongue out.
3. Bring the tip of the fibrescope as close as possible to the epiglottis and ask assistant to 'spray' lignocaine through the working channel.
4. Ensure that the suction line is kinked while the spray is done and for at least 30 seconds after the spray.
5. Patient will cough as soon as the local anaesthetic reaches the mucosa and the view will be temporarily lost.
6. After about 30 s advance the tip of the fibrescope under the epiglottis so that the vocal cords come in view.
7. Repeat the spray, this time directing the lignocaine on the vocal cords. You may need two, sometimes three, sprays until the movements of the cords become weaker.
8. Advance the fibrescope through the vocal cords, timing it during inspiration if possible.
9. The tracheal rings will come into view.
10. Advance the fibrescope towards the carina, being careful not to touch the tracheal wall and spray once more to anaesthetize the trachea and carina.
11. The endoscopy is now complete.

Railroading the tracheal tube

1. This is the most uncomfortable part of the procedure.
2. Administer more midazolam before beginning to railroad the tube.
3. Apply lubricating gel at the junction of the tube and the nose, but not on the tube to avoid it becoming very slippery.
4. Always tell patient at this stage that a tube is being passed, and that it may be uncomfortable.
5. Railroad the preformed nasal RAE tube through the nasopharynx and rotate it 90° anticlockwise to bring the tip of the tube anteriorly before advancing through the vocal cords.

Confirmation of tracheal tube position

1. Always confirm the position of the tube as the fibrescope is being pulled out of the tube.

2. Connect the tube to the breathing system and reconfirm tube position by movement of the bag and the presence of carbon dioxide on the monitor.
3. Administer the induction agent and muscle relaxant.

● **Example 2: Awake orotracheal fibreoptic intubation**

In the second example, a decision has been made to perform an awake orotracheal fibreoptic intubation using propofol target controlled infusion (TCI) for sedation and a translaryngeal injection for local anaesthesia. An Ovassapian airway will be used as a route guide (see Chapter 4). The '**preparing**' stage is similar to that described for nasotracheal intubation, except that an Ovassapian airway should be available and 5% lignocaine ointment to lubricate it.

Stage three: Performing awake orotracheal fibreoptic intubation

The steps of this stage are shown in Table 9.4.

Table 9.4   Performing orotracheal fibreoptic endoscopy and intubation

1. General
2. Preparing mouth and oropharynx
3. Performing translaryngeal injection (cricothyroid puncture)
4. Performing orotracheal endoscopy
5. Railroading the tracheal tube
6. Confirmation of tracheal tube position

General

1. Secure intravenous access.
2. Commence ECG and pulse oximetry monitoring and obtain blood pressure reading.
3. Sit up the patient on the trolley at 60°.
4. Administer midazolam 1 mg bolus and start TCI propofol at 1 µg/ml.

5. Administer supplemental oxygen with nasal cannula.
6. Constantly assess patient to ensure they respond to verbal commands.
7. Start topical anaesthesia when patient is relaxed but cooperative (usually 3–5 min).

Preparing mouth and oropharynx

1. Sit up patient on the trolley at 60°.
2. Ask the patient to open the mouth and administer 4–6 ml of 2% lignocaine gel to the back of the throat. Ask patient to gargle the solution in the mouth. Warn them that the taste will be bitter.
3. Gently suck the excess lignocaine and assess the gag reflex at the same time.
4. Instil more lignocaine gel until the gag reflex is sufficiently weak.

Performing translaryngeal injection (cricothyroid puncture)

1. Patient is supine with the head extended.
2. Identify the cricothyroid membrane.
3. After aseptic preparation, infiltrate the skin and subcutaneous tissue with 1% lignocaine.
4. Introduce a 22 G Venflon or Abbocath catheter (connected to a 5 ml syringe containing 2 ml of 4% lignocaine) into the cricothyroid membrane.
5. Direct the cannula caudad and aspirate for air when a give is felt.
6. Thread the cannula when air is aspirated and remove the needle and syringe.
7. Reattach the syringe to the cannula and confirm its correct placement by aspirating air.
8. Inject the solution after the end of normal expiration, always warning patient that they will cough.

Performing orotracheal endoscopy

1. Lubricate the surface of an Ovassapian airway with 5% lignocaine ointment and ask patient to suck, gradually pushing the airway to the back of the mouth at the same time until patient can tolerate it without gagging.
2. Apply gentle suction through the airway before you start.
3. Advance the insertion cord of the fibrescope (loaded with a flexometallic tube) through the Ovassapian airway.

4. The airspace is seen as soon as the tip of the fibrescope is out of the distal end of the airway and in the mouth.
5. Advance the fibrescope further to identify the epiglottis; negotiate the tip through the cords and into the trachea.
6. The SAYGO technique may be required if the transtracheal block is inadequate.

Railroading the tube

1. Gently insert the tube through the Ovassapian airway.
2. Continuously rotate the tube between the fingers to advance it (remember not to lubricate the outside of the tube or the fingers, otherwise rotation will be difficult).
3. Advance the tube until it is past the cords and in the trachea.

Confirmation of tracheal tube position

1. Always confirm the position of the tube as the fibrescope is being pulled out of the tube.
2. Connect the tube to the breathing system and reconfirm the tube position by the movement of the bag and the presence of carbon dioxide on the monitor.
3. Administer the induction agent and muscle relaxant.
4. The Ovassapian airway can be left *in situ* or peeled away from the tube.

Awake fibreoptic intubation in special situations

There are certain situations where special precautions are taken when performing awake fibreoptic intubation. Some of the conditions and their management are discussed.

■ The patient at risk of aspiration.
■ The pregnant patient.
■ The patient with unstable cervical spine.
■ The patient with critical upper airway obstruction.

● The patient at risk of aspiration

A rapid-sequence induction technique is generally used to prevent aspiration of gastric contents. This technique may not be appropriate in a patient who is at risk of aspiration and also has a difficult airway. Some examples include patients after trauma, pregnant patients, obese patients and those presenting for emergency surgery. Awake fibreoptic intubation is a safe option only when consideration is given to the following.

Premedication

Avoid sedative premedication. Prophylaxis for aspiration should be always prescribed. Ranitidine 150 mg and metoclopramide 10 mg orally if time permits or ranitidine 50 mg and metoclopramide 10 mg intravenously. Give 30 ml of 0.3 M sodium citrate prior to starting the procedure.

Administer scopolamine 0.2 mg IM or glycopyrrolate 0.2 mg intravenously. The antisialogogue action of anticholinergic agents is more beneficial in this situation than the risk of lowering the lower oesophageal sphincter tone.

Local anaesthetic technique

Some anaesthetists are concerned that local anaesthesia of the larynx obtunds the reflexes needed for protecting the airway. In a large series of 129 patients, both the translaryngeal injection technique and spray as you go (SAYGO) technique was effective and safe, with no evidence of regurgitation or aspiration in any patient [2]. A previous study found that an unprotected glottis might result from translaryngeal block [3]. There is evidence to suggest that local anaesthetic solution spreads on the superior aspect of the vocal cords after a translaryngeal block [4]. It has been suggested that topical anaesthesia of the larynx does not impair voluntary motor function of the vocal cords, such as coughing on request [5]. This allows the patient to protect himself/herself. SAYGO may be preferred because the interval between the topical anaesthesia and endoscopy is very small, and if aspiration occurred during endoscopy then it can be seen and action taken to prevent further aspiration and suck the gastric juice out with the fibrescope.

Technique of sedation

Sedation rather than topical anaesthesia of the larynx is more likely to cause laryngeal incompetence and risk of aspiration. If at all possible, awake fibreoptic intubation should be performed without sedation or it should be very carefully titrated.

Position of the patient

Gravity will prevent aspiration of gastric contents when fibreoptic endoscopy and intubation is performed in the sitting position or with the patient on the side and propped up.

● The pregnant patient (Figure 9.1)

A pregnant patient in whom a difficult intubation is anticipated may present for operative delivery. Most obstetric anaesthetists would prefer to use a regional technique when such a patient needs a caesarean section. However when regional anaesthesia is contraindicated or fails, most anaesthetists would choose to perform an awake fibreoptic intubation before induction of general anaesthesia [6]. The special considerations of performing an awake fibreoptic intubation in a pregnant patient are as follows:

1. Risk of aspiration.
2. Risk of bleeding with nasal intubation.
3. Effect of sedation on the neonate.

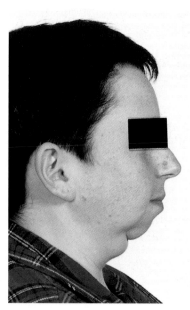

Figure 9.1 Pregnant patient with Still's disease in whom regional anaesthesia for caesarean section failed. An awake orotracheal fibreoptic intubation was performed before induction of general anaesthesia [9]

Risk of aspiration

All the precautions discussed when performing an awake fibreoptic intubation in a patient at risk of aspiration are relevant in the pregnant patient (see above).

Risk of bleeding with nasal intubation

The nasal mucosa is engorged in pregnancy, and bleeding during a nasal intubation may lead to a failed intubation and a compromised airway. The oral route is therefore preferred [7–9]. The nasal route may be indicated when oral fibreoptic intubation is contraindicated, e.g. swollen tongue [10]. Cocaine is relatively contraindicated for topical anaesthesia of the nasal cavity, as it may cause a decrease in utero placental blood flow. A mixture of 3 ml of 4% lignocaine and 0.25 ml of 1% phenylephrine applied with cotton-tipped applicators has been used [10]. Cocaine and phenylephrine both cause a decrease in uteroplacental blood flow, but the increase in systemic blood pressure with phenylephrine is less.

Effect of sedation on the neonate

Although awake fibreoptic intubation is possible without any sedation, it is difficult and unjustified to do so in a pregnant patient who is young and nervous. In most reports of awake fibreoptic intubation in pregnant patients, some sedation in the form of intravenous benzodiazepines and/or opioids has been administered. There is risk of respiratory depression and sedation in the neonate, but with modern paediatric resuscitation this should not be a reason for withholding sedation.

● The patient with unstable cervical spine

Direct laryngoscopy and intubation requires extension of the occiput on the atlas vertebra. This involves movement of at least the first three cervical vertebrae. There is controversy whether direct laryngoscopy results in spinal cord injury in the presence of an unstable spine. Firm evidence is lacking that spinal cord injury occurs due to positioning of the head and neck during laryngoscopy and intubation. In the case reports where this has been incriminated, other features such as hypotension and positioning of the patient for prolonged surgical periods may be more important [11]. Direct laryngoscopy and intubation while maintaining manual in-line traction is an accepted option in most cases. However, there are instances when awake intubation is preferred. These include a surgical policy of performing a brief neurological examination after intubation or when difficulty in intubation is anticipated, e.g. absent C1-C2 gap, trismus, micrognathia, surgical immobilization [12].

Awake fibreoptic intubation technique

It is desirable to perform endoscopy and intubation with the least coughing. Both the translaryngeal and SAYGO techniques result in coughing during their application. A technique using nebulized lignocaine may therefore be preferred. Adequate dose (6–8 ml of 4% lignocaine) and time (about 20 min) must be given for the nebulized lignocaine to work.

● The patient with critical airway obstruction

Awake fibreoptic intubation is indicated in the majority of patients with airway compromise (see Chapter 5). The morphology of the airway is abnormal but there are usually no or minimal signs of airway obstruction.

   A small group of patients with airway obstruction present with stridor, implying that the airway narrowing is at least 50%. An editorial has highlighted the issues of airway management in such patients [13].The airway management plan should include senior anaesthetists and surgeons, and each case should be judged individually. The site and extent of airway obstruction should be determined preoperatively. A primary technique and a back-up plan should be worked out in advance.

Upper airway obstruction

Causes: Perilaryngeal lesions of epiglottis, vocal cords, arytenoids and aryepiglottic folds.

If preoperative symptoms and nasendoscopy (by an ENT surgeon) suggest that intubation is not possible, the primary technique should be an awake tracheostomy. When there is moderate stridor and intubation is possible, one of the two options are possible. First, inhalation induction and direct laryngoscopy as a primary technique and the surgeon standing by to perform tracheostomy

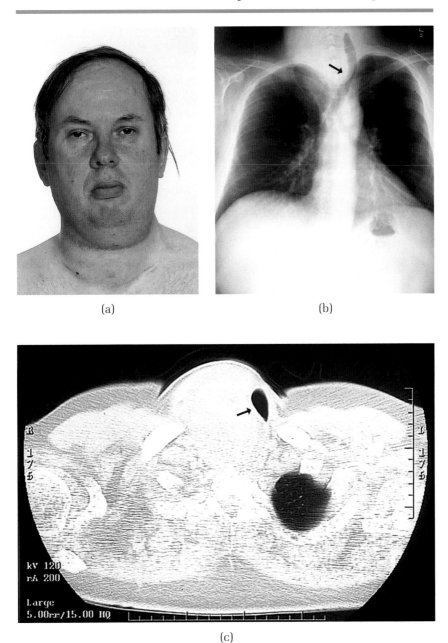

(a)

(b)

(c)

Figure 9.2 Patient with enlarged thyroid who presented with stridor (a). The trachea was deviated markedly to the left (b) and the site of maximum narrowing of the trachea was determined with MRI scans (c) (shown by arrows). An awake fibreoptic intubation was successfully performed with a 6.5 mm cuffed nasotracheal tube

under general anaesthesia if required (plan B). The place of the second option of awake fibreoptic intubation in this scenario is controversial. It may not be safe because of the risk of complete airway obstruction due to laryngeal spasm. This is provoked by local anaesthetic, blood or tumour fragments irritating the cords. The physical presence of the fibrescope in the airway may be sufficient to cause complete obstruction.

Mid-tracheal obstruction

Causes: e.g. retrosternal thyroid (Figure 9.2a–c).

The site of obstruction and its extent should be determined with the help of CT or MRI scans. In most cases a 6–7 mm tracheal tube can easily be railroaded through the obstruction. Awake fibreoptic intubation is a safe option, but should only be performed by an experienced endoscopist. The critical phase is passing the fibrescope and the tube past the narrow trachea.

Lower tracheal and bronchial obstruction

Causes: Mediastinal masses, vascular lesions.

The upper airway is usually normal and direct laryngoscopy is easy. There is danger of precipitating tracheal compression as soon as general anaesthesia is induced. For this reason, the ideal management of such patients is in a cardiothoracic centre with facilities for cardiopulmonary bypass facilities and expertise in rigid bronchoscopy.

● References

1. Koh KF, Hare JD, Calder I. Small tubes revisited. *Anaesthesia* 1998; **53:** 46–50.
2. Ovassapian A, Krejcie TC, Yelich SJ, Dykes MHM. Awake fibreoptic intubation in the patient at high risk of aspiration. *Br J Anaesth* 1989; **62:** 13–16.
3. Claaeys DW, Lockhart CH, Hinkle JE. The effect of translaryngeal block and Innovar on glottic competence. *Anesthesiology* 1973; **38:** 485–6.
4. Walts L, Kassity KJ. Spread of local anesthesia following upper airway block. *Arch Otolaryng* 1964; **81:** 77–9.
5. Mahajan RP, Murty GE, Singh P, Aitkenhead AR. Effect of topical anaesthesia on the motor performance of vocal cords as assessed by tussometry. *Anaesthesia* 1994; **49:** 1028–30.
6. Popat MT, Srivastava M, Russell R. Awake fibreoptic intubation skills in obstetric patients: a survey of anaesthetists in the Oxford region. *Int J Obst Anesth* 2000; **9:** 78–82.

7. Sidhu VS, Davies DWL. Fibreoptic oral intubation: a solution to difficult intubation in a parturient. *Anaesth Intens Care* 1995; **23:** 651.

8. D'Alessio JG, Ramanathan J. Fibreoptic intubation using intraoral glosso-pharyngeal nerve block in a patient with severe preeclampsia and HELLP syndrome. *Int J Obst Anesth* 1995; **4:** 168–71.

9. Popat MT, Chippa JH, Russell R. Awake fibreoptic intubation following failed regional anaesthesia for caesarean section in a parturient with Still's disease. *Eur J Anesthesiology* 2000; **17:** 211–14.

10. Mokriski BK, Malinow AM, Gray WC, McGuinn WJ. Topical nasophar-yngeal anaesthesia with vasoconstriction in preeclampsia-eclampsia. *Can J Anaesth* 1988; **35:** 641–3.

11. McLeod ADM, Calder I. Spinal cord injury and direct laryngoscopy – the legend lives on. *Br J Anaesth* 2000; **84:** 705–9.

12. Sidhu VS, Whitehead EM, Ainsworth QP, Smith M, Calder I. A technique of awake fibreoptic intubation. Experience in patients with cervical spine disease. *Anaesthesia* 1993; **48:** 910–13.

13. Mason RA, Fielder CP. The obstructed airway in head and neck surgery. *Anaesthesia* 1999; **54:** 625–8.

10

Difficult flexible fibreoptic intubation

- General and specific difficulties
- Difficult fibreoptic endoscopy
- Difficulty in railroading the tracheal tube
- Difficulty in removing fibrescope from the tracheal tube
- General points

● General and specific difficulties

Fibreoptic intubation is thought of as an impossible technique to master by many anaesthetists, who then perform it only occasionally, and find difficulty every time (don't want to do it). More commonly, an otherwise easy fibreoptic intubation is made difficult and this is usually due to poor technique and decision-making process (don't know how to do it). In experienced hands very few fibreoptic intubations are really difficult.

Failed fibreoptic intubation is the inability to pass the insertion cord in the trachea or railroad a tracheal tube. There were only five failures reported in a series of 413 nasotracheal fibreoptic intubations [1]. There is no agreed definition of 'difficult' fibreoptic intubation.

General difficulties with fibreoptic intubation are due to the following:

- Poor planning, e.g. inadequate patient and equipment preparation, inexperienced assistance.
- Wrong choice of technique, e.g. awake fibreoptic intubation in an uncooperative adult.
- Experience of the operator. Inexperience is one of the main causes of failed fibreoptic intubation [2].

A fibreoptic-guided tracheal intubation involves three stages: fibreoptic endoscopy, railroading the tracheal tube over the fibrescope and removing the fibrescope from the tracheal tube. **Specific difficulties** are related to the technical aspects of the three stages and may lead to failure of fibreoptic intubation. The aim of this chapter is to discuss the causes and practical solutions to the **specific** difficulties:

- Difficult fibreoptic endoscopy.
- Difficulty in railroading the tracheal tube.
- Difficulty in removing the fibrescope from the tracheal tube.

● Difficult fibreoptic endoscopy

During fibreoptic endoscopy the tip of the fibrescope is passed through the laryngeal inlet (the target) and into the trachea, allowing railroading of the tracheal tube. A good endoscopy technique involves negotiating the tip of the fibrescope under direct vision through the 'airspace' to reach this target, carefully avoiding contact with mucosa. Difficulties arise when vision is obscured by blood and secretions covering the objective lens, if the 'airspace' is obstructed or the target (laryngeal inlet) has been displaced due to abnormal anatomy. The causes of difficult fibreoptic endoscopy are summarized in Table 10.1.

Table 10.1   Causes of difficult fibreoptic endoscopy

Secretions or blood

Reduced airspace between the tip of epiglottis and posterior pharyngeal wall
General anaesthesia
Large floppy epiglottis
Oedema or cellulitis
Redundant mucosa (obesity, obstructive sleep apnoea)
Cervical spine deformity [3]
Supraglottic mass
Distorted airway anatomy (tumour, surgery, radiotherapy)

Deviated larynx

Reactive airway (inadequate anaesthesia)

The causes can be translated to the practical procedure of fibreoptic endoscopy and intubation as follows:

1. Inability to advance fibrescope through the nose (nasotracheal endoscopy).
2. Vision obscured by blood or secretions.
3. Inability to advance fibrescope due to reduction in airspace.
4. Able to see epiglottis but cannot get fibrescope through the cords.
5. Unable to see any airspace in pharynx/larynx.
6. Reactive airway (inadequate anaesthesia) – moving target.

Inability to advance the fibrescope through the nose (nasotracheal endoscopy)

This is most frustrating when it happens. Although the patency of the nasal cavity can be gauged from the history and examination, it is always good practice to introduce the tip of the fibrescope into both nostrils and choose the more patent one (Figure 10.1a,b). The practice of introducing the fibrescope 'blindly' in the nose can lead to obstruction, bleeding and discomfort in an awake patient. It may be helpful to 'size' the nostril by passing a well-lubricated, soft nasopharyngeal airway

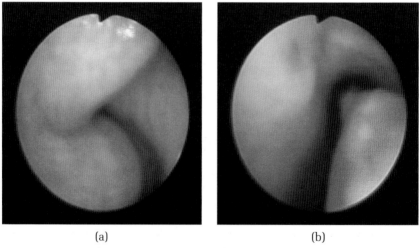

(a)   (b)

Figure 10.1   It is good practice to endoscope both nostrils before advancing the tip of the fibrescope in the nasal cavity. In this example the left nostril has virtually no space (a), while the right nostril is more patent and was chosen for intubation (b)

before endoscopy [4]. The orotracheal route of intubation is preferred in the presence of severe blockage.

Vision obscured by blood or secretions (Figures 10.2 and 10.3)

Blood interferes with the view of the airspace by its physical presence and also by internal reflections. Bleeding results from the fibrescope tip touching the mucosa (pink out or red out) and is prevented by a gentle, unhurried endoscopy technique where the tip is guided in the airspace under constant vision. Gentle suction will help to suck out blood, but endoscopy may have to

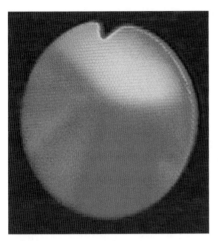 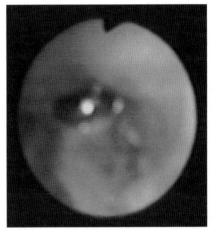

Figure 10.2 Bleeding in the upper airway makes endoscopy difficult and can be prevented by a gentle technique

Figure 10.3 Secretions make fibreoptic endoscopy difficult. Thick secretions clog the lens and thin secretions cause internal reflection

be abandoned in cases of massive haemorrhage. A fibrescope with a larger suction channel or direct laryngoscopy may then be preferred. During an unanticipated difficult intubation, repeated attempts at direct laryngoscopy may result in bleeding, making it impossible to use the fibrescope. In these situations, fibreoptic intubation should be used early in the airway plan.

Secretions may be thin or thick. Secretions cause vision difficulties both directly and by increasing internal reflections. Antisialogogue premedication is useful in drying the mouth before fibreoptic intubation [5,6]. Direct gentle suction of the oropharynx before fibreoptic endoscopy is useful because the suction capacity of the fibrescope is weak. If secretions are thick, the fibrescope should be withdrawn and external suction used to clear them. The awake patient can be asked to swallow the secretions. High-flow oxygen through the working channel of the fibrescope helps to clear secretions and improves vision [7]. Fogging of the lens will also interfere with vision and can be avoided by inserting the fibrescope tip in warm water or cleaning it with an alcohol wipe before endoscopy.

Inability to advance fibrescope due to reduction in airspace

General anaesthesia reduces the muscle tone in the upper airway so that the soft palate, tongue and epiglottis fall backwards onto the posterior pharyngeal wall (Figure 10.4.a) [8]. Inappropriate

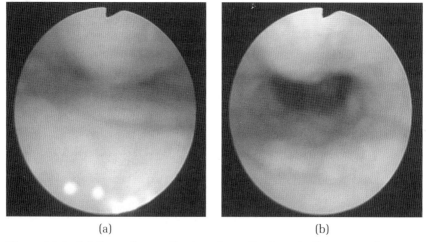

(a)   (b)

Figure 10.4   (a) General anaesthesia reduces the tone in the upper airway so that the soft palate, tongue and epiglottis fall backwards on the posterior pharyngeal wall. (b) A jaw thrust manoeuvre usually opens the airway

sedation will also have the same effect. Little or no airspace is then left in the oropharynx for manoeuvring the tip of the fibrescope and the view will be obscured by tissue (white out). Pathological causes that reduce the airspace are from within the airway and include a floppy epiglottis, oedema or cellulitis of the pharyngeal tissues (Figure 10.5a,b) or from pressure without, including deformity of the cervical spine [3] and supraglottic mass.

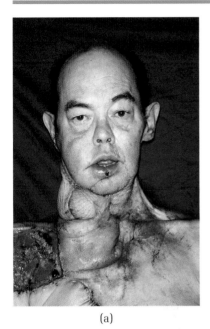

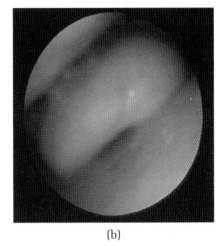

(a)   (b)

Figure 10.5 Difficult fibreoptic endoscopy: (a) reduction in airspace in a patient with multiple scarring from surgery and radiotherapy; (b) fibreoptic endoscopy revealed a swollen, oedematous epiglottis. Endoscopy was successful after the patient was sat up and was made to take deep breaths, thus opening the airspace

One or more of the following manoeuvres opens the airspace and helps in negotiating the tip of the fibrescope towards the glottis:

- Asking an assistant to provide jaw thrust (Figure 10.4b).
- Neck extension (cf. direct laryngoscopy) by removing the pillow or placing a pillow under the shoulder [9].
- Tongue protrusion with a gauze piece [10].
- External pressure on the larynx to move it backwards [11].
- Combining fibreoptic and direct laryngoscopy to lift the epiglottis/tongue [12,13].
- Changing the position of patient to lateral or sitting (if patient is awake).
- Asking the awake patient to sniff, swallow or breathe deeply (if patient is awake).

The angle required to reach the larynx during orotracheal endoscopy is more acute than during nasotracheal endoscopy and there is a tendency of the tip of the fibrescope to hit the base of the tongue. This is avoided by using fibreoptic airway aids (e.g. Berman airway, Ovassapian airway), which displace the tongue away from the posterior pharyngeal wall, permit the concentric insertion of the fibrescope and also keep the tip of the fibrescope in the midline (see Chapter 4).

Able to see epiglottis but cannot get fibrescope through the cords

Distorted anatomy around the laryngeal structures will prevent the fibrescope from entering the glottis. The tip deflection of an intubating fibrescope is usually limited to 120° and the field of vision to 90°. Basically you can see where you want to go but cannot get there. It is worth trying all the above manoeuvres, but if the problem is due to fixed tissues, then railroading may also be difficult despite a successful endoscopy. There are two guide wire techniques, that may be considered.

Anterograde wire technique

Only the distal 2 cm of the insertion cord 'bends' with the movement of the control lever. The idea of the anterograde wire technique is to increase this length to allow the tip of the fibrescope to enter the glottis. Any guide wire that is at least 110 cm long and able to pass through the suction channel of an intubating fibrescope can be used. A dedicated wire set is available (e.g. Cook retrograde wire), but a cardiac catheter wire that is generally available in most hospitals will suffice (e.g. 150 cm and 0.098 mm diameter). The practical steps of the technique are as follows:

1. Lubricate a suitable guide wire and pass it through the working channel of the fibrescope so that its tip is just short of the tip of the fibrescope.
2. Perform endoscopy and bring the tip of the fibrescope as near the vocal cords as possible.
3. Ask assistant to feed the wire and gently manipulate the tip of the fibrescope so that the wire moves with tip deflection and enters through the vocal cords (Figure 10.6a,b).
4. Pass a sufficient length of wire in the trachea and then railroad the insertion cord of the fibrescope over it and confirm its position.

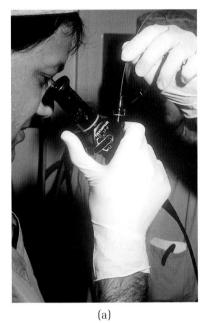
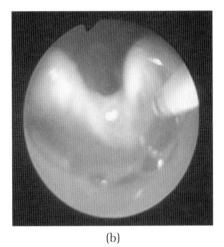

(a)   (b)

Figure 10.6   Anterograde wire technique. Bring the tip of the fibrescope as near to the larynx as possible and ask an assistant to feed a wire through the working channel (a) until it comes out at the distal end, negotiate it through the cords and into the trachea (b). Railroad the fibrescope over the wire and into the trachea

5. Remove the wire and railroad a tracheal tube over the fibrescope and check its position.

If this technique fails, try a retrograde guide wire technique (see below).

Unable to see any airspace in pharynx/larynx

All the manoeuvres described to open the airspace may be tried. Deep breathing may be useful in an awake patient and an air bubble may be seen, indicating an airspace. It is worth guiding the fibrescope tip in any hole and hope that it may be the correct one! If everything fails, try a retrograde guide wire technique.

Retrograde guide wire technique

1. Patient is supine with the head extended.
2. Place a suitable 20 G cannula through a cricothyroid or transtracheal puncture and direct it towards the vocal cords.

3. Pass a guide wire through the cannula and grasp it with a forceps in the mouth.
4. Gently pull the wire out of the mouth making sure enough length is left at the neck end.
5. Feed the tip of the wire coming out of the mouth into the distal end of the working channel of the fibrescope and thread it upwards until it comes out from the working channel port.
6. Under vision, railroad the fibrescope over the guide wire until the tip of the fibrescope passes through the vocal cords and the tip of the cannula is seen
7. Withdraw the cannula and wire slowly and under constant vision.
8. Ensure that a sufficient length of the fibrescope is in the trachea.
9. Railroad a tracheal tube over the fibrescope and check its position.

Reactive airway (inadequate anaesthesia) – moving target

In general, fibreoptic intubation is easier to perform in an awake patient because all the problems of general anaesthesia are avoided. A cooperative patient will also assist by sniffing, taking deep breaths and positioning himself/herself. Difficulties arise if topical anaesthesia of the airway is inadequate, resulting in excessive movements of the larynx accompanied by coughing, retching and laryngospasm. Additional lignocaine sprayed through the suction channel of the fibrescope will usually solve the problem. A small dose of intravenously administered opioid may also depress the cough reflex. Adequate sedation must be ensured before railroading the tube as this is the most unpleasant part of the procedure. The laryngeal reflexes may be reactive if fibreoptic endoscopy and intubation are performed under light general anaesthesia, especially in a spontaneously breathing patient (see Chapter 6).

● **Difficulty in railroading the tracheal tube**

Difficulties in railroading the tracheal tube are caused by its tip impinging on the laryngeal structures, especially at the arytenoids [14]. They are related to the size, the flexibility and design of the tube and the technique of railroading (see Chapter 6).

Size of tube

It is difficult to railroad a tracheal tube through the vocal cords if the gap between the fibrescope and the tube is big. Tracheal tubes of 6–7 mm are ideal, as they will snugly fit on the insertion cord of an intubating fibrescope (4 mm). If bigger tubes are required, fibrescopes with an insertion cord diameter of 5–6 mm may be used [15]. Another method of overcoming the problem is to interpose a 5 mm uncuffed tracheal tube (Figure 10.7) [16] or an Aintree Intubating Catheter [17] between the tracheal tube

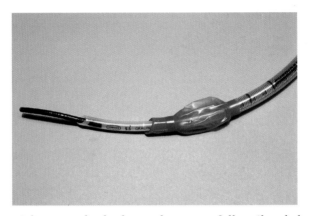

Figure 10.7   A larger tracheal tube can be successfully railroaded over a 4 mm fibrescope by interposing a smaller uncuffed tracheal tube between the fibrescope and the larger tube

and the fibrescope. By protruding the smaller tube or catheter beyond the larger tracheal tube, the access to the trachea is gained in two smaller steps, thereby preventing its tip impinging on the arytenoids.

Flexibility and design of tube

The flexibility of the tube determines the ease with which it conforms to the insertion cord of the fibrescope. Flexometallic tubes were railroaded 19/20 times compared with 7/20 successes with a regular tracheal tube at first pass [18]. The design of the tip of the tracheal tube also determines the success rate of railroading. A newly designed tube with a conical, tapered tip without a bevel was superior to a standard tube during both orotracheal and nasotracheal intubation [19]. The tube is not available commercially. The intubating laryngeal mask airway (ILMA) tube with a tapered tip was more successful when compared with an ordinary Portex tube for orotracheal intubation [20]. For nasal intubation, a previously warmed, north-facing preformed tube (e.g. RAE Mallinckrodt) achieves a high success rate of railroading when it is rotated 90° clockwise (see below).

Technique of railroading

The hold-up of the advancement of the tracheal tube during railroading occurs due to the resistance of the laryngeal structures. The right arytenoid is the commonest site for the tube to 'hold up' in the neutral position, i.e. when the tip of the tracheal tube is to the right-hand side and the bevel is facing the left side [21]. A 90° counterclockwise rotation of the tube will bring the tip of the tube anteriorly, permitting it to enter the trachea without resistance [22]. When hold-up occurs, withdraw the tube slightly, maintain a clear airway (jaw thrust) and then rotate the tube 90° anticlockwise. Flexometallic tracheal tubes are easily railroaded when they are continuously rotated between the fingers while advancing them over the fibrescope [23]. It is important *not* to lubricate the outside of the tube or your fingers when using this technique. A rigid laryngoscope blade may also be useful to elevate the epiglottis and facilitate railroading [24].

● Difficulty in removing fibrescope from the tracheal tube

Difficulties arise if the fibrescope has not been lubricated before mounting the tracheal tube on it. Some anaesthetists introduce a tracheal tube in the pharynx and then pass the fibrescope through it (tube-first method). This may lead to the fibrescope tip passing through the Murphy eye rather than the distal end of the tube, causing difficulty in its removal [25,26]. The preferred technique is inserting the fibrescope under direct vision into the trachea and railroading the tube over it.

Checking position of the tracheal tube

The position of the tube must be confirmed when the fibrescope is being removed from the tube, as accidental oesophageal intubation can occur due to movement of the fibrescope during railroading. The position must be rechecked by presence of end tidal carbon dioxide *after* the fibrescope is withdrawn, to ascertain that the tube has not come out during withdrawal of the fibrescope.

● General points

1. Direct laryngoscopy may be easy when fibreoptic intubation is difficult in the presence of secretions and blood.
2. Details of a difficult fibreoptic intubation must be documented in the patient's notes.
3. A patient in whom a difficult fibreoptic intubation has been documented should be intubated awake.
4. Transtracheal ventilation is an option to ventilate a patient during a difficult fibreoptic intubation [27].

● References

1. Ovassapian A, Yelich SJ, Dykes MHM, Brunner EE. Fiberoptic nasotracheal intubation – incidence and causes of failure. *Anaesth Analg* 1983; **62:** 692–5.
2. Ovassapian A. Fibreoptic tracheal intubation in adults. In: Ovassapian A ed. *Fibreoptic Endoscopy and the Difficult Airway*, 2nd edn, pp. 72–103. Lippincott-Raven, Philadelphia, 1996.
3. Ranasinghe DN, Calder I. Large cervical osteophyte – another cause of difficult flexible fibreoptic intubation. *Anaesthesia* 1994; **49:** 512–14.
4. Edens ET, Sia RL. Flexible fiberoptic endoscopy in difficult intubations. *Annals Otol Rhinol Laryngol* 1981; **90:** 307–9.
5. Brookman CA, Teh Pin H, Morrison LM. Anticholinergics improve fibreoptic intubating conditions during general anaesthesia. *Can J Anaesth* 1997; **44:** 165–7.
6. Watanabe H, Lindgren L, Rosenberg P, Randall T. Glycopyrronium prolongs topical anaesthesia of the oral mucosa and enhances absorption of lignocaine. *Br J Anaesth* 1993; **70:** 94–5.
7. Rosen DA, Rosen KR, Nahrworld ML. Another use for the suction port on the pediatric flexible bronchoscope. *Anesthesiology* 1986; **65:** 116.
8. Nandi PR, Charlesworth PR, Taylor SJ, Nunn JF, Dore CJ. Effect of general anaesthesia on the pharynx. *Br J Anaesth* 1991; **66:** 157–62.
9. Mason RA. Learning fibreoptic intubation: fundamental problems. *Anaesthesia* 1992; **47:** 729–31.
10. Archdeacon J, Brimcombe J. Anterior traction of the tongue – a forgotten aid to awake fibreoptic intubation. *Anaesth Intens Care* 1995; **23:** 750–57.
11. Bond A. Assisting fibreoptic intubation. *Anaesth and Intens Care* 1992; **20:** 247–8.
12. Johnson C, Hunter J, Ho E, Bruff C. Fibreoptic intubation facilitated by rigid laryngoscope. *Anesth Analg* 1991; **72:** 713.
13. Dennehy KC, Dupuis JY. Fibreoptic intubation in the anaesthetised patient. *Can J Anaesth* 1996; **43:** 197–8.

14. Cossham PS. Difficult intubation. *Br J Anaesth* 1985; **57:** 239.
15. Hakala P, Randell T. Comparison between two fibrescopes with different diameter insertion cords for fibreoptic intubation. *Anaesthesia* 1995; **50:** 735–7.
16. Marsh NJ. Easier fibreoptic intubations. *Anesthesiology* 1992; **76:** 860–61.
17. Atherton DPL, O'Sullivan E, Lowe D, Charters P. A ventilation– exchange bougie for fibreoptic intubations with the laryngeal mask airway. *Anaesthesia* 1996; **51:** 1123–6.
18. Brull SJ, Wiklund R, Ferris C, Connelly NR, Ehrenwerth J, Silverman DG. Facilitation of fiberoptic orotracheal intubation with a flexible tracheal tube. *Anaesth Analg* 1994; **78:** 746–8.
19. Jones HE, Pearce AC, Moore P. Fibreoptic intubation. Influence of tracheal tube design. *Anaesthesia* 1993; **48:** 672–4.
20. Lucas DN, Yentis SM. A comparison of the intubating laryngeal mask tracheal tube with a standard tracheal tube for fibreoptic intubation. *Anaesthesia* 2000; **55:** 358–61.
21. Schwartz D, Johnson C, Roberts JA. A maneuver to facilitate flexible fiberoptic intubation. *Anesthesiology* 1989; **71:** 470–71.
22. Hughes S, Smith JE. Nasotracheal tube placement over the fibreoptic laryngoscope. *Anaesthesia* 1996; **51:** 1026–8.
23. Thorin D, Rosselet P, Ravussin P, Spuhler S. Impact of the endotracheal tube on glottic and supraglottic structures during orotracheal fibreoptic intubation. *Br J Anaesth* 1995; **74(suppl):** A42.
24. Katsnelson T, Frost EAM, Farcon E, Goldiner PL. When the endotracheal tube will not pass over the flexible fibreoptic bronchoscope. *Anesthesiology* 1992; **76:** 151–2.
25. Ovassapian A. Failure to withdraw flexible laryngoscope after nasotracheal intubation. *Anesthesiology* 1985; **63:** 124–5.
26. Calder I. When the endotracheal tube will not pass over the flexible fiberoptic bronchoscope. *Anesthesiology* 1992; **77:** 398.
27. Cooper DW, Long GT. Difficult fibreoptic intubation in an intellectually handicapped patient. *Anesth Int Care* 1992; **20:** 227–9.

11

Paediatric fibreoptic intubation

Airway difficulties in the paediatric population may arise from congenital or acquired lesions. History and examination of previous notes may point to a diagnosis, especially of the various syndromes that may be associated with a difficult airway. Details of previous airway management may also be found.

A physical examination helps in predicting airway difficulty. Some anatomical features associated with difficult airway in adults may also be present in children. These include micrognathia (e.g. Pierre Robin syndrome, Treacher Collins syndrome, Goldenhar's syndrome), short neck (Down's syndrome, Klippel–Feil syndrome), large tongue (Down's syndrome) or severe hydrocephalus. Other uncommon congenital anomalies associated with a difficult airway are also described [1].

Tests of predicting difficult intubation in adults (e.g. Mallampati test) may be appropriate in cooperative children, although their usefulness has not been formally evaluated.

Fibreoptic intubation is a useful technique of securing the airway when difficulties are anticipated with mask ventilation and/or tracheal intubation.

● Fibreoptic equipment

The availability of special ultrathin fibrescopes with a bending tip has made a big impact on the use of fibreoptic intubation in

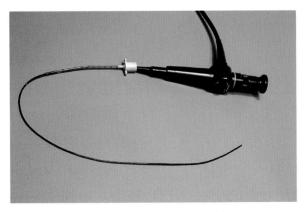

Figure 11.1   Olympus LF-P paediatric intubating fibrescope. A 2.5 mm tracheal tube can easily be loaded over its insertion cord which has a diameter of 2.2 mm. There is no working channel in this fibrescope

paediatrics. Examples are the Olympus LF-P (2.2 mm diameter) or Pentax FI-7BS (2.4 mm diameter). A tracheal tube with a 2.5 mm ID can easily be passed over the Olympus LF-P fibrescope (Figure 11.1). A bending section at the distal end is provided, but there is no working channel. This makes it impossible to perform suction, insufflate oxygen or instil local anaesthetic when using these fibrescopes. Most investigators have found the ultrathin fibrescopes useful for intubating neonates or infants[2] and for teaching fibreoptic intubation in children[3]. Other investigators have felt that the vision was good but the fibrescope easily curled up in the pharynx and was difficult to manipulate through the cords, resulting in a 12% failure[4]. They commented that the fibrescopes were 'whippy'. Perhaps the real reasons for failure were that the fibrescope was used in older children using a spontaneously breathing technique (see below).

Adult intubating fibreoptic laryngoscopes (e.g. Olympus LF-2, 4 mm diameter or Pentax FI-10BS, 3.5 mm diameter) can be used in children in whom the size of the required tube is 5 mm or larger. The adult fibrescope has also been used for indirect fibreoptic intubation techniques in smaller children (see below).

● Airway aids

Airway aids maintain ventilation or act as a conduit for the fibrescope during oral endoscopy (see Chapter 4). A paediatric endoscopy mask (VBM®) is available for maintaining ventilation. An ordinary disposable facemask can be adapted with a corrugated tube and a silicon diaphragm for the same purpose [5]. There is a lack of airway aids that act as a conduit for the fibrescope, although an ingenious method of splitting an ordinary Guedel airway is described for this purpose [6]. Paediatric Berman airways are only suitable for older children. The best airway aid for paediatric fibreoptic intubation is a laryngeal mask airway (LMA). It acts as a conduit, maintains ventilation during endoscopy and avoids trauma to the airway, and is particularly useful in the presence of blood and secretions. It has been used for both nasal and oral fibreoptic intubation in spontaneously breathing and paralysed patients. Its placement and fibreoptic intubation in an awake infant has been described [7].

● Fibreoptic intubation techniques

All the fibreoptic intubation techniques described for adult patients can be used in paediatric patients. Techniques in both awake and anaesthetized patients are used via the orotracheal or nasotracheal route.

It is important to understand some anatomical and physiological factors, especially in neonates and infants, that may influence the techniques of fibreoptic intubation. The anatomical landmarks are small, with very little distance for manipulation, and the structures appear quickly at the tip, requiring immaculate techniques. The neonatal epiglottis is angular, long and stiffer than the adult epiglottis. The larynx is more cephalad and the vocal cords are angled more anteriorly. It is therefore vital to keep the tip of the fibrescope in the midline and there may be difficulty in getting it past the cords. The narrowest part of the child's airway is at the level of the cricoid and force must not be used to railroad tracheal tubes.

Profuse salivation in children makes it mandatory to use antisialogogue premedication routinely. When the airway is traumatized, oedema and spasm quickly result in desaturation. Fibreoptic techniques should therefore be considered early in the airway management plan. Care must also be taken to obtund laryngeal reflexes with deep general anaesthesia, suxamethonium or local anaesthetic when performing intubation in the spontaneously breathing patient.

● Fibreoptic intubation under general anaesthesia

Direct technique

In this technique, the fibrescope is manipulated into the trachea and the tracheal tube is railroaded over it. Tracheal tubes with diameters as small 2.5 mm ID can be railroaded over ultrathin fibrescopes. The adult fibrescope is used for railroading tubes larger than 5 mm ID. Both nasotracheal and orotracheal routes can be used in spontaneously breathing or paralysed patients.

The fibrescope can be kept in the midline during orotracheal intubation by tongue traction with gauze or an atraumatic forceps. A useful technique is to ask an assistant to provide jaw thrust and for the anaesthetist to rest the hand holding the insertion cord on the patient's face, thus giving leverage to insert the tip of the fibrescope in the midline directly [8].

Indirect techniques

The direct technique cannot be used to intubate children requiring tracheal tubes smaller than 5 mm ID if an ultrathin paediatric fibrescope is unavailable. An adult intubating fibrescope is used to visualize the vocal cords, but intubation is not directly performed over it. Instead a wire is inserted through the working channel of the fibrescope into the trachea and intubation performed by railroading the tube over the guidewire [9,10]. A larger tube may not railroad satisfactorily over a small guide wire, when the technique is modified by first railroading a wire stiffener [11], a tube exchanger or ureteric catheter to provide stiffness. This two-stage technique is time consuming and may risk the patient desaturating during airway manipulation. The LMA is used to overcome these problems [12] and its use as an airway aid is described below.

Indirect technique using LMA (Figure 11.2)

The LMA acts as a conduit for the fibrescope and also helps to maintain ventilation during manipulations of the fibrescope. The technique can be used in paralysed or spontaneously breathing patients. The steps of the technique are as follows:

1. Insert a LMA in the usual fashion.
2. Confirm ventilation through it after connection to the breathing circuit with a 15 mm fibreoptic swivel self-sealing connector to facilitate delivery of oxygen and inhalation agent (Figure 11.2a).

3. Pass a 110 cm guide wire (e.g. Cook retrograde or a cardiac catheter wire) through the working channel of the fibrescope until its tip is just short of the tip of the fibrescope.
4. Pass the fibrescope through the swivel connector into the LMA and negotiate its tip though the bars of the LMA, under the epiglottis, to visualize the vocal cords (Figure 11.2b).

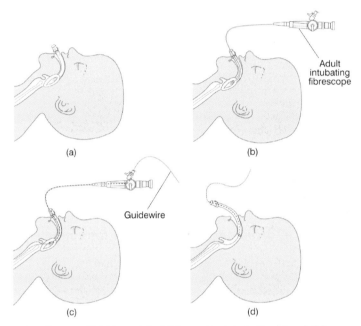

Figure 11.2 Steps of LMA-assisted fibreoptic intubation in children using an adult fibrescope and guide wire: (a) insert a LMA and connect it to a breathing system with a fibreoptic swivel connector (not shown); (b) pass the tip of an adult fibrescope (Olympus LF-2) through the LMA bars until the vocal cords are visualized; (c) pass a guide wire through the working channel of the fibrescope until its tip passes through the vocal cords; (d) remove the LMA and fibrescope, and railroad a suitable tracheal tube over the guide wire

5. Ask an assistant to push the wire through the vocal cords and into the trachea (Figure 11.2c).
6. Remove the LMA and fibrescope, leaving the wire in the trachea.
7. Railroad a suitable size tracheal tube over the wire (Figure 11.2d).

If the size of the tube is large, a small tube exchanger, wire stiffener or ureteric catheter is first railroaded over the wire to stiffen it and the tube subsequently railroaded over it.

Other techniques are described below, but are not commonly used.

Fibreoptic observation technique

The fibrescope passed through one nostril is used to visualize the passage of the tube through the other nostril and into the larynx [13].

Retrograde technique with fibreoptic guidance

A guide wire is passed through the cricothyroid membrane in a retrograde fashion and is grasped in the mouth. It is then threaded up the distal end of the fibrescope, which is already loaded with an endotracheal tube. The fibrescope is then passed through the cords over the guide wire and the tube is railroaded over the fibrescope [14]. This technique is useful when there are a lot of secretions in the oropharynx making visualization difficult.

Combined use of direct laryngoscopy and fibreoptic intubation

The combined technique is useful when the upper airway is obstructed and cannot be opened with the usual manoeuvres or in the presence of blood and secretions. The laryngoscope blade helps to lift the tongue and epiglottis, making visualization of the cords easier [15].

● Awake fibreoptic intubation

Awake fibreoptic intubation is feasible in children, although most anaesthetists choose a technique under general anaesthesia. In the older child a good explanation of the technique with support from the parents and appropriate premedication will ensure cooperation. Premedication must always include an antisialogogue. The other aspects of preparation for awake intubation, including equipment checks, monitoring and supplemental oxygenation, are similar to adults (see Chapter 7). The principles of conscious sedation and local anaesthesia of the upper airway are also similar but certain important considerations are discussed.

Conscious sedation

The popular combination of fentanyl and midazolam may be used, especially in older children. In the younger child, ketamine is a good agent and offers the following advantages:

- Hypnotic and analgesic.
- Suitable for children of all age groups.
- Preserves spontaneous ventilation.
- Preserves patent airway.
- Can be administered by many routes (IV, IM, oral, rectal and intranasal).
- Emergence reactions are uncommon in children.

Ketamine increases salivary secretions, but with antisialogogue premedication this is not a problem.

Topical anaesthesia

All the techniques described for achieving local anaesthesia of the airway in adults can be used in children (see Chapter 8). Topical application is the most popular method. A lot of children have experience of using nebulizers for asthma and this is a good technique to use. Care must be taken not to exceed the maximal dose of 4 mg/kg of lignocaine. This equates to 0.2 ml/kg of 2% solution or 0.1 ml/kg of 4% solution.

● Service and training

The most important factor in determining the success of fibreoptic intubation in paediatric patients is the experience of the anaesthetist. He/she should not only be competent in anaesthetizing paediatric patients, but also skilled in using fibreoptic and ancillary equipment. This combination may only be possible in big teaching centres. There is a move in the UK to perform paediatric surgery in dedicated centres and it is likely that expertise will be concentrated there. A child with a difficult airway, presenting for elective surgery, should benefit from this expertise. These centres should also take on the responsibility of training future consultants. In smaller hospitals, one consultant may not possess the combined expertise in paediatric anaes-thesia and fibreoptic intubation and in this situation two or more consultants should jointly manage the patient.

Paediatric fibreoptic intubation techniques should be learnt by anaesthetists with an interest in paediatric anaesthesia. The principles of learning should involve a structured training programme (see Chapter 2). It is important that a paediatric anaesthetist is skilled in performing fibreoptic intubation in adults before practising in children. Once they are skilled in adults, practice on paediatric patients with normal airways is highly desirable before managing patients with difficult airways. The efficacy and safety of fibreoptic intubation training in children with normal airway under general anaesthesia has been confirmed [16]. Fibreoptic intubation takes longer than conventional laryngoscopy but has no additional complications [3].

● References

1. Wheeler M, Ovassapian A. Pediatric fibreoptic intubation. In: Ovassapian A ed. *Fibreoptic Endoscopy and the Difficult Airway*, 2nd edn, pp. 105–15. Lippincott-Raven, Philadelphia, 1996.
2. Finer NN, Muzyka D. Flexible endoscopic intubation of the neonate. *Pediatr Pulmonol* 1992; **12**: 48–51.
3. Roth AG, Wheeler M, Stevenson GW, Hall SC. Comparison of a rigid laryngoscope with the ultrathin fibreoptic laryngoscope for tracheal intubation in infants. *Can J Anaesth* 1994; **41**: 1069–73.
4. Wrigley SR, Black AE, Sidhu VS. A fibreoptic laryngoscope for paediatric anaesthesia: a study to evaluate the use of the 2.2 mm Olympus (LF-P) intubating fibrescope. *Anaesthesia* 1995; **50**: 709–12.
5. Frei FI, Ummenhofer W. A special mask for teaching fiber-optic intubation in pediatric patients. *Anesth Analg* 1993; **76**: 450–61.
6. Wilton NCT. Aids for fiberoptically guided intubation in children. *Anesthesiology* 1991; **75**: 549–50.
7. Johnson CM, Sims C. Awake fibreoptic intubation via a laryngeal mask in an infant with Goldenhar's syndrome. *Anaesth Intens Care* 1994; **22**: 194–7.
8. Wheeler M. The difficult pediatric airway. In: Hagberg C ed. *Handbook of Difficult Airway Management*, pp. 257–300. Churchill Livingstone, Philadelphia, 2000.
9. Howardy-Hansen P, Berthelsen P. Fibreoptic nasotracheal intubation of a neonate with Pierre Robin syndrome. *Anaesthesia* 1988; **43**: 121–2.
10. Scheller JG, Schulman SR. Fiber-optic bronchoscopic guidance for intubating a neonate with Pierre Robin sequence. *J Clin Anesth* 1991; **3**: 45–7.
11. Stiles CM. A flexible fiberoptic bronchoscope for endotracheal intubation of infants. *Anesth Analg* 1974; **53**: 1017–19.
12. Hasan MA, Black AE. A new technique for fiberoptic intubation in children. *Anaesthesia* 1994; **49**: 1031–3.
13. Alfery DD, Ward CF, Harwood IR, Mannino FL. Airway management for a neonate with congenital fusion of the jaws. *Anesthesiology* 1979; **51**: 340–42.

14. Audanaert SM, Montgomery CL, Stone B, Akins RE, Lock RL. Retrograde-assisted fiberoptic tracheal intubation in children with difficult airways. *Anesth Analg* 1991; **73:** 660–64.
15. Haas JE, Tsueda K. Direct laryngoscopy with the aid of a fiberoptic bronchoscope for tracheal intubation. *Anesth Analg* 1996; **82:** 438.
16. Erb T, Marsch SU, Hampl KF, Frei FJ. Teaching the use of fiberoptic intubation for children older than two years of age. *Anesth Analg* 1997; **85:** 1037–41.

12

Flexible fibreoptic instruments: applications in anaesthesia and intensive care

Mansukh Popat and Stuart Benham

- Tube placement and position check
- Tube change
- Diagnostic/therapeutic endoscopy
- Difficult extubation

The clinical application of flexible fibreoptic instruments has escalated since their introduction in medicine in the early 1950s. Initially slow to embrace the technology, anaesthetists now use flexible fibrescopes for a variety of reasons (Table 12.1). These uses can be applied in the operating theatre, intensive care unit (ICU) and in the accident and emergency department.

● Tube placement and position check

Tracheal tube placement

The main use of flexible fibreoptic instruments is for tracheal intubation in patients with normal and difficult airways. This is the main subject of this book and has been extensively discussed in previous chapters.

Checking tracheal tube position

When used for intubation, fibreoptic endoscopy offers a quick and most definitive method of confirming the position of the tube in the trachea. Fibreoptic endoscopy can also provide a safe, reliable

Table 12.1   Clinical applications of flexible fibreoptic instruments in anaesthesia and intensive care

Tube placement and position check
Tracheal tubes
Double lumen endobronchial tubes
Endobronchial blockers
Nasopharyngeal airway
Nasogastric tube
Percutaneous tracheostomy

Tube change
Oral to nasal route
Nasal to oral route
Single lumen to double lumen or vice versa

Diagnostic/therapeutic Endoscopy
Upper airway
Bedside bronchoscopy

Difficult extubation

and quick method to check tube position in adults and children [1,2] in the ICU instead of chest X-rays. Checking tube position with X-rays has certain disadvantages including the time delay, difficulty in identifying the tip, movement of the patient, increased risk of disconnection and exposure to radiation [3,4].

Technique of checking tracheal tube position with a fibrescope

1. Attach a 15 mm fibreoptic swivel connector to the tracheal tube.
2. Administer 100% oxygen via a breathing system.
3. Advance the fibrescope into the tracheal tube and place its tip at the carina (Figure 12.1a).
4. Mark this position on the fibrescope with a firm hold of the thumb and index finger (first mark = carina level) (Figure 12.1b).
5. Withdraw the fibrescope slowly until the edge of the tube is seen (Figure 12.1c).
6. The junction of the swivel connector and fibrescope is the second mark (second mark = tube level) (Figure 12.1d).

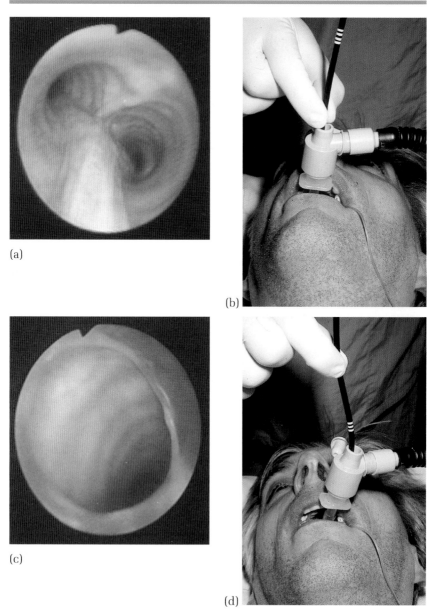

(a)

(b)

(c)

(d)

Figure 12.1 Checking the tracheal tube position. Pass a fibrescope into a tracheal tube and advance its tip to the carina (a). Mark this position on the fibrescope with a firm hold of thumb and finger as the 'first mark' (b). Withdraw the fibrescope until the edge of the tube is seen (c). The junction of the fibrescope and swivel connector (d) is the 'second mark'. The difference between the first and second marks is the distance between the edge of the tube and carina

7. The distance between the first and second marks is the distance between the tip of the tube and the carina. This distance is between 2 and 4.5 cm in adults.

Obstruction in the lumen of the tube can also be identified and the tube withdrawn if endobronchial intubation has resulted. Dynamic assessment of the tube position in flexion and extension of the head and in the prone or sitting position during surgery can also be made.

Double lumen endobronchial tube (DLEBT) placement and position check

Traditionally, DLEBTs have been placed with direct laryngoscopy and their position checked by auscultation of the lungs. A number of studies have highlighted the high incidence of malposition by blind methods and the superiority of fibreoptic visualization [5]. A recent national confidential enquiry into perioperative deaths (NCEPOD) reported that 30% of deaths were related to DLEBTs during oesophagogastrectomy. Most were managed by senior anaesthetists and none used the fibrescope to confirm the position of the tube, either before or during surgery, even when the tube was evidently incorrectly placed [6]. It is recommended that a fibrescope should be used to place a DLEBT accurately in all patients and that this should be rechecked after patient positioning and during the procedure to maintain optimal positioning and for sputum clearance [5]. Fibreoptic-guided placement of a DLEBT in an awake patient with a difficult airway has also been reported [7].

Equipment

A tracheal intubating fibrescope (e.g. Olympus LF-2, 4 mm) will pass through the tracheal and bronchial lumens of DLEBT larger than 35 FG. Dedicated fibrescopes with insertion cord diameter of 3.1 mm are available for placement of double lumen tubes (e.g. Olympus LF-DP and Pentax FI-9BS). These fibrescopes will pass through most DLEBTs.

Fibreoptic techniques for DLEBT placement

The fibreoptic techniques of DLEBT placement, including the bronchial and tracheal endoscopy views, have been extensively reviewed [8]. A modified description of the techniques described by Ovassapian follows [9].

Technique of fibreoptic-assisted left-sided DLEBT placement

A properly placed left-sided DLEBT should have its tracheal lumen 2–3 cm above the carina. The tip of the bronchial lumen should not occlude the left upper lobe bronchus and the bronchial cuff should be confined to the inside of the left main bronchus.

1. Induce anaesthesia and paralyse patient.
2. At direct laryngoscopy, introduce the DLEBT through the larynx, rotated 90° clockwise so that the bronchial tip is anterior.
3. Once the tracheal cuff is past the glottis, rotate the tube to the left and inflate the tracheal cuff.
4. Institute mechanical ventilation.
5. Introduce the fibrescope through the bronchial lumen of the tube and check the length and patency of the left main bronchus.
6. Place the tip of the fibrescope a few millimetres above the level of the left upper lobe bronchus.
7. Deflate the tracheal cuff, hold the fibrescope stationary and advance the tube into the left main bronchus until the tip of the tube just passes the tip of the fibrescope.
8. Inflate the tracheal cuff to secure the tube and advance the fibrescope beyond the bronchial lumen to visualize the orifice of the left upper lobe bronchus and ensure that the tube is not impinging on it.
9. Remove the fibrescope and pass it down the tracheal lumen of the DLEBT. Visualize the carina, the opening of the right main bronchus and the bronchial cuff (blue). If the bronchial cuff is not seen, withdraw the tube slightly.
10. Inflate the bronchial cuff under direct vision of the fibrescope.
11. Clamp the tracheal lumen connector limb and open its suction port to air. Patient is now being solely ventilated through the bronchial lumen; inflate the cuff until there is an airtight seal.
12. Remove the clamp from the tracheal lumen connector limb. Deflate the tracheal tube cuff and reinflate it with the minimal leak technique.

Technique of checking position of left-sided DLEBT

Some anaesthetists prefer to insert the DLEBT blindly, check its position clinically and finally confirm it with a fibrescope as follows:

1. Pass the fibrescope in the tracheal lumen of the DLEBT until its tip comes out in the trachea.
2. Visualize the carina, the opening of the right main bronchus and the cuff of the endobronchial lumen as a blue crescent (Figure 12.2a).

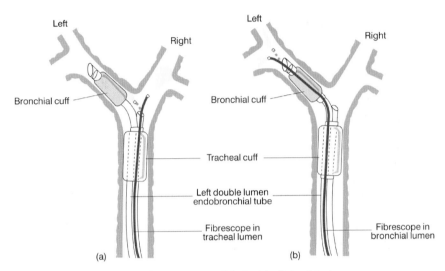

Figure 12.2 Checking the position of left-sided double lumen endotrachial tube (DLEBT) with a fibrescope. (a) Advance the fibrescope in the tracheal lumen of the DLEBT. Visualize the carina and opening of the right main bronchus. The edge of the blue endobronchial cuff is just visible. (b) Advance the fibrescope into the bronchial lumen of the DLEBT. Visualize the bifurcation of the left main bronchus and opening of the left upper lobe bronchus

3. Remove the fibrescope from the tracheal lumen and pass it through the bronchial lumen until it comes out at the end.
4. Visualize fully the bifurcation of the left main bronchus and the opening of the left upper lobe bronchus (Figure 12.2b).

Technique of fibreoptic-assisted right-sided DLEBT placement

Proper placement of the right DLEBT is more difficult than the left side due to the short and variable length of the right main stem bronchus.

1. Place the DLEBT in the trachea and inflate the tracheal cuff.
2. Introduce the fibrescope through the bronchial lumen of the right DLEBT and into the right main stem bronchus to check its patency and length.
3. Withdraw the fibrescope into the lumen of the bronchial lumen of the DLEBT and rotate it through 90° clockwise to position its tip at the proximal end of the ventilation window in the bronchial cuff.
4. Advance the tube and the fibrescope into the right main stem bronchus until the opening of the right upper lobe orifice appears through the ventilation cuff window.
5. Advance the tube further so that the distal edge of the window passes 1–2 mm beyond the distal border of the right upper lobe bronchial orifice.
6. Now advance the fibrescope until its tip is at the midpoint of the ventilation window, allowing visualization of the right upper lobe bronchial lumen.
7. Rotate and advance the fibrescope toward the distal end of the tube, allowing visualization of the right lower lobe bronchial openings.
8. Remove the fibrescope from the bronchial lumen, insert it into the tracheal lumen and visualize the carina, left main bronchus and the bronchial cuff of the right DLEBT.

Technique of checking right-sided DLEBT

Some anaesthetists prefer to insert the DLEBT blindly and check it clinically. The fibrescope is used to confirm the position as follows:

1. Pass the fibrescope in the tracheal lumen of the DLEBT until its tip is in the trachea.
2. Visualize the carina, the opening of the left main bronchus and the blue cuff of the bronchial lumen of the DLEBT (sometimes difficult to see with right DLEBT) (Figure 12.3a).
3. Remove the fibrescope from the tracheal lumen and pass it into the bronchial lumen until its tip is in the middle of the ventilation slot in the bronchial cuff.
4. A deflection of the tip should visualize the opening of the right upper lobe bronchus. Advance it further to visualize segmental bronchi (Figure 12.3b).
5. Withdraw the tip from the upper lobe bronchus and into the bronchial lumen of the DLEBT.

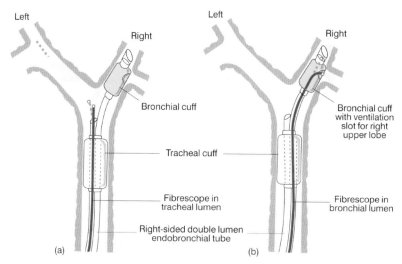

Figure 12.3 Checking the position of right-sided double lumen endobronchial tube (DLEBT) with a fibrescope. (a) Advance the fibrescope in the tracheal lumen of a right DLEBT and visualize fully the carina and opening of the left main bronchus. The blue endobronchial cuff may just be seen. (b) Advance the fibrescope tip in the bronchial lumen until the middle of the ventilation slot is reached and deflect it to fully visualize the opening of the right upper lobe bronchus. Withdraw the fibrescope in the bronchial lumen and advance it further to visualize the right lower lobe bronchus

6. Advance it forward to check the patency of the right lower lobe bronchus (Figure 12.3b).

Fibreoptic-assisted placement and checking of endobronchial blockers

The operated lung or its segment can be isolated with the help of endobronchial blockers. These can be inserted with fibreoptic guidance and their position checked. The Univent blocker is a modified tracheal tube with a built-in channel for a movable blocker that can be guided by fibreoptic visualization in the appropriate lumen of the main or segmental bronchi. After verifying the position of the blocker, a balloon is inflated and its position secured with a stopper at the proximal end.

Nasopharyngeal airway placement and position check

It is crucial to choose the proper size of a nasopharyngeal airway to relieve airway obstruction. After preparation of the nasal cavity with local anaesthetic and vasoconstrictor, a nasopharyngeal airway can be guided over a fibrescope, avoiding trauma. Its correct position in relation to the tongue and nasopharynx is easily assessed with the fibrescope [10].

Nasogastric tube placement and position check

Nasogastric tubes are usually placed blindly in awake or anaesthetized patients. Its placement in the anaesthetized patient can be facilitated by a simple technique using a fibrescope.

A fibrescope loaded with an uncut, uncuffed 7 mm tracheal tube is loaded on a fibrescope, which is deliberately inserted in the oesophagus via the nose. The fibrescope is removed from the tube and a nasogastric tube is passed through the tracheal tube into the oesophagus. Alternatively, if the use of a tracheal tube is not desired, then a guide wire can be passed in an anterograde fashion in the oesophagus, the fibrescope is removed and a nasogastric tube railroaded over the guide wire. When there is doubt about the position of a nasogastric tube, fibrescope endoscopy can confirm that placement is in the oesophagus and not through the glottis.

Fibreoptic-assisted percutaneous tracheostomy

Percutaneous tracheostomy (PT) is now a routine bedside technique of providing tracheal access instead of a standard surgical tracheostomy. The technique of serial dilatation is commonly used [11]. The practical steps of the technique are described elsewhere [12]. The complication rate is low and may include tube displacement, haemorrhage, false passage, subcutaneous emphysema and pneumothorax [13]. A fibreoptic-assisted technique is recommended to minimize and detect these complications [14,15]. The fibrescope can be used during placement of a PT during the following steps:

1. To provide illumination for entry of needle and catheter into the tracheal site.
2. To check position of needle entry site.
3. To verify the position of the guide wire.
4. To check the position of the tracheostomy tube at insertion.
5. To confirm satisfactory position of the tracheostomy tube by passing the fibrescope through it.

● Tube change

Oral to nasal route or vice versa; single lumen to double lumen tube or vice versa

It may be necessary to change tracheal tubes for a number of reasons that include tube blockage, cuff leak, surgical access and size. In most cases this can be achieved with direct laryngoscopy. In some patients, a fibreoptic technique offers additional safety [16]. These include patients with a difficult airway, in those with a risk of complications such as epistaxis, unstable spine or haemodynamic instability.

Fibreoptic-assisted changing of oral to nasal tube
(Figure 12.4)

1. Patient is anaesthetized and preferably paralysed.
2. Prepare nasal cavity with local anaesthetic and vasoconstriction.
3. Insert the fibrescope loaded with a tracheal tube into the nostril (Figure 12.4a).
4. Perform endoscopy under direct vision from nose to pharynx while assistant performs jaw thrust.
5. Identify the oral tube entering the larynx (Figure 12.4b).
6. Manipulate the tip of the fibrescope anterior to the tube, in the space between the tube and the anterior commissure.
7. Deflate the cuff of the oral tube when the tip of the fibrescope is past the cords and the cuff is seen.
8. Advance the fibrescope in the trachea beside the original tube until the carina is seen (Figure 12.4c).
9. Remove the oral tube and quickly railroad the nasal tube and check its position (Figure 12.4d).

The advantages are a minimal apnoea time and prevention of tracheal soiling with maximum possible control of airway. An alternative method is to pass a nasal tube in the nasopharynx first and then introduce the fibrescope through it. The rationale for success of these techniques is that there is always some space between the tube and the vocal cords, usually anteriorly, and that the diameter of the adult trachea is about 2 cm, so that a fibrescope (4 mm) can easily lie adjacent to the original tube.

A similar technique is used to change an oral tube to another oral tube or a nasal to an oral tube.

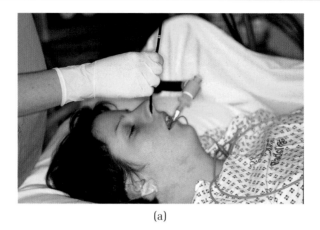

(a)

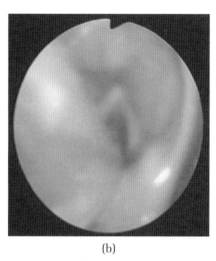

(b)

Figure 12.4 Fibreoptic-assisted changing of oral to nasal tracheal tube: (a) advance the fibrescope loaded with a nasotracheal tube into the nasal cavity; (b) identify the oral tube entering the larynx – manipulate the tip of the fibrescope past the oral tube into the trachea and deflate its cuff.

It may not be possible to insert the fibrescope beside a DLEBT, when it needs to be changed to a single lumen tube. In this case the tip of the fibrescope (loaded with a tracheal tube) is brought near the larynx, the cuff of the DLEBT is deflated and it is gently withdrawn. The fibrescope is quickly passed into the trachea and the tube railroaded over it. Secretions may obstruct the view and the oropharynx should be thoroughly sucked out before and during the procedure.

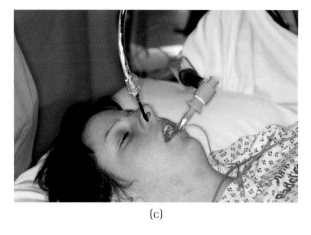

(c)

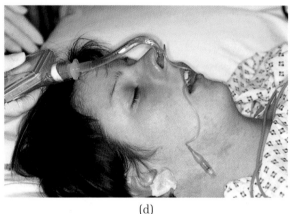

(d)

Figure 12.4 (*continued*)   (c) railroad the nasal tube after quickly removing the oral tube; (d) the oral tube has now been changed to a nasal tube

● Diagnostic/therapeutic endoscopy

Upper airway endoscopy

Fibreoptic endoscopy is useful for evaluation of the upper airway in a variety of conditions. Some include burns, trauma and obstruction due to infection, tumour or foreign body [17]. It has also been used to assess the function of the vocal cords following thyroid surgery [18]. Anaesthetists contemplating this use must be skilled and experienced in all aspects of fibreoptic endoscopy.

Bedside diagnostic and therapeutic bronchoscopy

This procedure refers to the bedside bronchoscopy performed in the ICU or in the recovery room for diagnostic and limited therapeutic purposes. The examination is usually limited to the proximal bronchial segments.

Some indications of diagnostic bronchoscopy are to establish the causes of hypoxaemia, haemoptysis and unexplained hypercapnia. Its clinical applications in the theatre or ICU include lung collapse, pneumonia and trauma. At the time of performing a bronchoscopy, limited therapeutic interventions such as vigorous bronchial toilet to remove mucous plugs, blood clots or tenacious secretions can be performed to expand the collapsed segments. The procedure should only be undertaken by those experienced in this area. The detailed aspects of application of fibreoptic bronchoscopy in the ICU are beyond the scope of this chapter and have been reviewed [17,19].

A 15 mm fibreoptic bronchoscopic swivel connector is attached to the tracheal tube and 100% oxygen administered via the breathing system. Full monitoring is established and ideally another anaesthetist should monitor and administer drugs to the patient. Care must be taken in presence of severe hypoxaemia, worsening hypercapnia, haemodynamic instability, recent myocardial infarct, pulmonary hypertension, unstable cardiac rhythm and coagulopathy. Complications of bedside bronchoscopy may include tachycardia, hypertension and arrhythmias. Hypoxaemia and hypoventilation can result due to increased resistance to breathing or due to coughing and bronchospasm. The patient must be sedated with opioids and laryngeal reflexes obtunded with local anaesthetics or muscle relaxants to prevent the effects of bronchoscopy. The bronchoscope narrows the lumen of the tracheal tube causing pressure-limited reduction in tidal volume, increasing both the inspiratory and expiratory resistance. Passing the bronchoscope in the bronchi of a non-diseased lung may worsen any V/Q mismatch. The following recommendations allow a safe bronchoscopy to be performed.

Recommendations for diagnostic/therapeutic bronchoscopy

- 100% inspired oxygen.
- Ensure sedation and paralysis.
- Monitor patient parameters.
- Monitor ventilatory parameters.
- Consider volume-cycled ventilation.

- Consider size of tracheal tube, ideally 8 mm.
- Suction for short periods only.
- Check post-procedure chest X-ray.

● Difficult extubation

A flexible fibrescope can be an invaluable aid in determining the cause of difficulty in tracheal extubation (e.g. a stitch) and can assist in reintubation using a tube change technique [20].

● References

1. Whitehouse AC, Klock LE. Evaluation of endotracheal tube position with fibreoptic intubation laryngoscope. *Chest* 1975; **68**: 848.
2. Vigneswaran R, Whitfield JM. The use of a new ultra-thin fiberoptic bronchoscope to determine endotracheal tube position in the sick newborn infant. *Chest* 1981; **80**: 174–7.
3. O'Brien D, Curran J, Conroy J, Bouchier-Hayes D. Fiberoptic assessment of tracheal tube position. A comparison of tracheal tube position as estimated by fiberoptic bronchoscope and by chest X-ray. *Anaesthesia* 1985; **40**: 73–6.
4. Yezerski J, Arnold BL, Sachtello CR. Technique to locate the end of an endotracheal tube. *Crit Care Med* 1984; **12**: 600–601.
5. Pennefather SH, Russell GN. Placement of double lumen tubes – time to shed light on an old problem. *Br J Anaesth* 2000; **84**: 308–10.
6. Sherry K. Management of patients undergoing oesophagectomy. In: Gray AJG, Hoile RW, Ingram GS, Sherry KM eds. *The Report of the National Confidential Enquiry into Perioperative Deaths 1996/1997*, pp. 57–61. NCEPOD, London, 1998.
7. Patane PS, Sell BA, Mahla ME. Awake fiberoptic endobronchial intubation. *J Cardiothoracic Anesth* 1990; **4**: 229–31.
8. Slinger PD. Fiberoptic bronchoscopic positioning of double-lumen tubes. *J Cardiothoracic Vascul Anesth* 1989; **3**: 486–96.
9. Ovassapian A. *Fibreoptic-Aided Bronchial Intubation*. In: Ovassapian A ed. *Fibreoptic Endoscopy and the Difficult Airway*, 2nd edn, pp. 117–37. Lippincott-Raven, Philadelphia, 1996.
10. Stoneham MD. The nasopharyngeal airway. Assessment of position by fibreoptic laryngoscopy. *Anaesthesia* 1993; **48**: 575–80.
11. Ciaglia P, Graniero KD. Percutaneous dilational tracheostomy. Results and long term follow up. *Chest* 1992; **101**: 464–7.
12. Soni N. Percutaneous tracheostomy: how to do it. *Br J Hosp Med* 1997; **57**: 339–45.
13. Schwann NM. Percutaneous dilational tracheostomy: anesthetic considerations for a growing trend. *Anesth Analg* 1997; **84**: 907–11.
14. Marelli D, Paul A, Manolidis S et al. Endoscopic guided percutaneous tracheostomy: early results of a consecutive trial. *J Trauma* 1990; **30**: 433–5.

15. Dulgerov P et al. Percutaneous or surgical tracheostomy: a meta analysis. *Crit Care Med* 1999; **27:** 1617–25.
16. Rosenbaum SH, Rosenbaum LH, Cole RP et al. Use of the flexible fiberoptic bronchoscope to change endotracheal tube in critically ill patients. *Anesthesiology* 1981; **54:** 169–70.
17. Ovassapian A. Fibreoptic airway endoscopy in critical care. In: Ovassapian A ed. *Fiberoptic Endoscopy and the Difficult Airway*, 2nd edn, pp. 157–84. Lippincott-Raven, Philadelphia, 1996.
18. Akhtar TM. Laryngeal mask airway and visualisation of vocal cords during thyroid surgery. *Can J Anaesth* 1991; **38:** 140–3.
19. Spring C, McCririck A. The fibre-optic bronchoscope in the ICU. *Br J Intens Care* 1999; **9:** 14–22.
20. Popat MT, Dravid RM, Watt-Smith SR. Use of the flexible intubating fibrescope for tracheal re-intubation in a patient with difficult extubation. *Anaesthesia* 1999; **54:** 359–61.

Appendix: Flexible fibreoptic and ancillary equipment distributor list in the United Kingdom

The following information was correct at the time of going to press.

Olympus® flexible fibreoptic endoscopes
Light sources
Camera and closed circuit television monitor
KeyMed Ltd
KeyMed House
Stock Road
Southend-on-Sea
Essex SS2 5QH
Tel.: 01702 616333
Fax: 01702 465677
Website: www.keymed.co.uk

Pentax® flexible fibreoptic endoscopes
Light sources
Camera and closed circuit television monitor
Pentax UK LTD
Pentax House
Heron Drive
Langley,
Slough SL3 8PN
Tel.: 01753 792792
Fax: 01753 792794
Website: www.pentax.co.uk

'Oxford' Fibreoptic teaching box
Pharmabotics Ltd
The Gate House
Nyewood Industrial Estate
Rogate
West Sussex GU31 5HA
Tel: 01730 818282
Fax: 01730 818282
Website: www.pharmabotics.com

Perasafe® peracitic acid disinfectant
Antec International
Windham Road
Chilton Industrial Estate
Suffolk CO10 6XD
Tel.: 01787 377305
Fax: 01787 375391
Website: www.antec.org.uk

Berman Intubating Airway
Vital Signs Inc
Sussex Business Village
Lake Lane
Barrington
Barnham PO22 0AL
Tel.: 01243 555300
Fax: 01243 555400

Ovassapian Airway
The Kendall Company (UK) Ltd
2 Elmwood
Chineham Business Park
Crockford Lane
Basingstoke
Hampshire RG24 8WG
Tel.: 01256 708880
Fax: 01256 708071

VBM Bronchoscope Airway
VBM Endoscopy Mask
Freelance Surgical Promotions
Unit 2, Olympia House
Beaconsfield Road
St George
Bristol BS5 8ER
Tel.: 0117 9414147
Fax: 0117 9414848

Aintree Intubation Catheter
Endotracheal tube changers
Wires for anterograde/retrograde intubation
Cook Critical Care
Monroe House
Lechworth
Hertfordshire SG6 1LN
Tel.: 01462 473100
Fax: 01462 473190

Laryngeal Mask Airway
Intubating Laryngeal Mask Airway
Intavent Orthofix
Barney Court
Cordwallis Park
Maidenhead
Berkshire SL6 7BZ
Tel.: 01628 594500
Fax: 01628 789400
Website: www.intaventorthofix.com

Cuffed Oropharyngeal Airway (COPA)
Tracheal and endobronchial double lumen tubes
Mallinckrodt Medical (UK) Limited
10 Talisman Business Centre
London Road
Bicester OX6 0JY
Tel.: 01869 322700
Fax: 01869 321890
Website: www.mallinckrodt.com

Fibreoptic Swivel connector
Chimney Airway
Gum elastic bougie
Tracheal and endobronchial double lumen tubes
SIMS Portex Limited
Hythe
Kent CT21 6JL
Tel.: 01303 260551
Fax: 01303 265560
Website: www.portex.com

Index